T0176349

PARTIAL TRUTHS

PARTIAL TRUTHS

How Fractions Distort Our Thinking

JAMES C. ZIMRING

Columbia University Press
New York

Columbia University Press
Publishers Since 1893
New York   Chichester, West Sussex
cup.columbia.edu

Library of Congress Cataloging-in-Publication Data
Names: Zimring, James C., 1970- author.
Title: Partial truths : how fractions distort our thinking / James C. Zimring.
Description: New York, NY : Columbia University Press, 2022. |
    Includes bibliographical references and index.
Identifiers: LCCN 2021039876 (print) | LCCN 2021039877 (ebook) |
    ISBN 9780231201384 (hardback) | ISBN 9780231554077 (ebook)
Subjects: LCSH: Critical thinking. | Cognitive psychology. | Suicide victims.
Classification: LCC BF441 .Z55 2022 (print) | LCC BF441 (ebook) |
    DDC 153.4/2—dc23/eng/20211104
LC record available at https://lccn.loc.gov/2021039876
LC ebook record available at https://lccn.loc.gov/2021039877

Columbia University Press books are printed on permanent and
    durable acid-free paper.
Printed in the United States of America

Cover design by Henry Sene Yee

To Kim, Alex, and Ruby
who make my fraction whole ∾

CONTENTS

ACKNOWLEDGMENTS

Starting with a blank page and ending with a published book is no small process, and it inevitably entails the contributions and encouragement of a great many people—such is certainly the case with this book. I have babbled incessantly to friends and colleagues (the colleagues also being friends) on the underlying themes and concepts in this book for years, and they all have my thanks for the patient feedback and dialog, including the suggestion of specific examples that have been incorporated into the text. In particular, I would like to state my heartfelt appreciation to Steven Spitalnik, Patrice Spitalnik, Angelo D'Alessandro, Katrina Halliday, Chance John Luckey, Krystalyn Hudson, Eldad Hod, Heather Howie, Janet Cross, Jacqueline Poston, Karolina Dziewulska, and Ariel Hay. I would like to specifically recognize Ryan D. Tweney, who kindly served as a sounding board and mentor in cognitive psychology, as well as a friend, and who very sadly passed away during the writing of this manuscript—I will ever miss the ability to pick up the phone and learn from you.

I am particularly indebted to Lee McIntyre who has kindly and graciously mentored me as a developing author, both in general and also regarding critical feedback on the thoughts and concepts in this book. I am also indebted to the academic feedback from Cailin O'Connor, Mark Edward, Karla McLaren, Carla Fowler, David Zweig, and Steven Lubet. I would also like to thank the peer-reviewers who kindly volunteered their time to review and provide critical feedback for the text—while you will ever remain anonymous to me, you have my thanks—it is a significantly stronger book as a result of your constructive criticism.

From the first draft of this book to the finished product, I have had the great fortune to receive the assistance of many capable individuals, including Al Desetta, Miranda Martin, Zachary Friedman, Robyn Massey, Leah Paulos, Marielle Poss, Noah Arlow, and Ben Kolstad. Special thanks to Jeffrey Herman for support and encouragement.

Above all others, I am grateful to my family, for their never-ending support, love, and encouragement.

PARTIAL TRUTHS

INTRODUCTION

We humans are awfully fond of ourselves. From antiquity to the present day, a considerable part of Western scholarship in philosophy, psychology, biology, and theology has tried to explain how something as splendid and marvelous as humans could ever have come into being. For theologians of the Abrahamic religions, humans were created in an image no less grandiose than that of God. Philosophers as far back as antiquity have categorized humans as superior to all other animals, clearly set apart by the ability to reason. Aristotle described humans as a rational animal.[1] Rene Descartes felt that animals were like automated machines that were not able to think; only humans had the capacity to reason. Of course, such scholars knew that humans behave irrationally at times, perhaps even often, but they explained this behavior as a failure to suppress the animalistic tendencies that lurk within us. Humans were the only animals with the ability to reason, whether or not they always did so. To develop our minds and learn the discipline to give our reason control over our actions was accomplished by the study of philosophy, which was the road to a life well lived by achieving an inner harmony of the mind that lined up with the intrinsic harmony of the universe. In modern terms, whether human reason is a gift from the gods (or one God), or the result of natural selection does not matter—what seems clear is that the human ability to reason exceeds that of all other animals on Earth and sets us apart from the beasts.[2]

Contrary to the long-standing narrative of our self-proclaimed splendor, in just the past 50–60 years, the field of cognitive psychology has described an ever-increasing litany of errors that human cognition makes in observation, perception, and reasoning. Such "defects" are most prevalent for certain types of problems and in particular circumstances, but they are unequivocally present. Of course, all people do not think and act the same way. Cognition varies from person to person, and factors such as particular experience, genetic and environmental variation, and cultural context influence how a given person's mind may work. Nevertheless, all humans have some version of a human brain in their skull, which uses a general cognitive apparatus that we all carry. When I write of human cognition, I am referring to how humans think on average—that is, not how a specific human may think, but rather how many (or most) do.

Our new understanding of human cognition is nothing short of shocking. Over and over again, in a variety of different ways, cognitive psychologists have demonstrated that (under certain specific conditions), humans consistently fail even simple tasks in reasoning and logic. Perhaps more concerning, humans have defects in seeing and understanding the world around us as it "really" is.[3] Forget that we may not be able to use the facts of the world to reason logically, we cannot even observe many of the facts to begin with. Finally, and perhaps most troubling, humans have remarkably poor insight into our own thinking, often being entirely unaware of the way we process information and the effects of different factors on these processes.

This does not mean we lack insight into our minds; we actually perceive quite a lot about how our minds work. Humans have little problem reflecting on why we have reached certain conclusions, evaluating what may have influenced us, and explaining the reasons and reasoning behind the choices we make—it is just that we often get it wrong. As error prone as humans are in observing and reasoning, we are just as bad in our mental self-assessment. Even when we are bumbling about making errors, we tend to think we are right. If nothing else, at least cognitive psychology has explained why humans have spent so much time trying to explain how splendid humans are—it is in our nature to misperceive ourselves in a favorable light.

Two fundamental questions will be considered in this book. First, how can we really understand, in depth, what kinds of errors we make and how those errors affect our internal thinking and our perception of the external world? To shed light on human thinking, this book focuses on the concept of a fraction to explore the fundamental form underlying a variety of human errors.

Second, if humans really are so cognitively flawed, if we observe incorrectly, and if we think illogically, then how can we explain how effective humans are at using reason to make tools, solve problems, develop advanced technologies, and basically take over the world?

Setting aside the debate of whether human advancements are good or bad—that is, whether we are making progress toward some laudable end or just destroying the world and each other—it is difficult to deny that humans have made massive technological progress and solved many extremely complex problems. How can such an error-prone cognition accomplish such a task? Has cognitive psychology just got it all wrong, or can we find some other explanation? These issues will be formally addressed in chapter 11, although they will be lurking in the background throughout the book. The main focus of this book, however, is to describe one particular form that underlies many errors, to analyze its properties so we can better understand it, to learn to recognize it, to investigate its manifestations in the real world, and to consider strategies to avoid such errors.

The Form of the Errors

Yogi Berra, the famed baseball player and manager who had a talent for witticism (intentional or not), once went into a restaurant and ordered a pizza. When the chef behind the counter asked him if he wanted it cut into four or six pieces, he answered, "you better cut the pizza into four pieces because I'm not hungry enough to eat six." Berra was also quoted as saying, "Baseball is 90 percent mental; the other half is physical." Both of these statements are funny because they violate intuitive rules regarding how fractions work.

In this book, we explore how human cognition handles problems that fit the form of a fraction, including risks, odds, probabilities, rates, percentages, and frequencies. It is hard to navigate modern life without encountering and using these concepts. Exploring how fractions work and how we understand (and misunderstand) them will help us see why many of our deep-seated intuitive thought processes, however they work neurologically, are susceptible to particular errors. It also reveals that what are errors in some settings can offer great advantages in others. Overall, understanding fractions can help us understand ourselves.

Counterintuitive Properties of Rates, Frequencies, Percentages, Probabilities, Risks, and Odds

Although simple in concept, the prosaic fraction has complex nuances. As such, we are susceptible to both innocent misunderstanding and purposeful manipulation of fractions. We wield issues like percentages and risk as common notions, and often we do so effectively. We might not notice, however, when we misunderstand them, likely because concepts such as probabilities and frequencies apply to populations. Human cognition evolved in the setting of small nomadic groups of people with basically anecdotal experiences—not in the context of analyzing sets of data that reflect populations.[4]

This likely explains why humans favor anecdotal information to high-quality population-based data, even though for many purposes, the latter is profoundly more powerful than the former, if (and only if) analyzed properly.[5]

The result is that common sense is commonly mistaken, in particular when applied to types of information that we did not evolve to handle. This likely explains why erroneous thinking can "feel right" by our intuitions—we don't recognize that we are analyzing different kinds of information. But there is good news. When humans are exposed to explanations and demonstrations that reveal they may be wrong, they have the capacity to remedy their conclusions, if not their underlying instincts. The bad news is that humans are much less adept at modifying their thinking to spot and prevent errors on their own. Even when we discover what errors can occur, and learn to recognize the circumstances in which they do so, the right answer may still "feel" incorrect. Eons of evolution are not so easily overcome.

A Few Caveats

In writing this book, an inescapable irony has been ever present in my mind. I strive to give a balanced view and consider alternative arguments, but I nevertheless am selective in the evidence I present. Book length, author bandwidth, and reader attention span are limited. In other words, in writing a book about noticing only a fraction of information in the world, I can present only a fraction of the available evidence—both for and against this concept. I am mindful that this book is written in a Western philosophical and intellectual tradition. I am strongly committed to avoiding notions of cognitive or cultural imperialism; however, I am a product of my culture and biased by my perspective. Finally, I wrote this book using a version of the human brain (although some who know me might deny that claim). So, by my own arguments, I am prone to misperceive the fraction about misperceiving the fraction, and to be quite unaware that I have done so. To the extent that the interactionist model of human reasoning is correct (as detailed in chapter 11), at least I know that my arguments will be vetted through the dispute and disapproval of others. My experience as a scientist and author makes me confident that, to the extent that anyone takes notice, there will be no shortage of disputation and criticism. In the greatest traditions of scientific practice, I welcome this intellectually, if not also emotionally.

Organization and Goals of This Book

Part 1 of the book defines and explains a series of circumstances that can lead to misunderstanding as a result of the form information or ideas take (that can be represented by fractions). I use examples from both the controlled setting of the laboratory and also the real world to describe these processes and to understand their nuances. Part 2 builds on part 1 to further explore manifestations in the real world and in particular contexts. The areas explored range from politics to the criminal justice system, to alternative and New Age beliefs, to the argument for intelligent design of the universe, and even to the hard sciences. This wide range of areas is explored because the cognitive processes discussed are present whenever human minds think, and as such, they manifest in whatever humans think about.

Part 3 explores how cognitive errors also can be highly advantageous and arguably essential to the ability of humans to figure things out. These considerations bear directly on the apparent contradiction between how error prone humans are and how successful we have been in advancing our understanding and technology. The impulse to automatically think that we should eradicate what we perceive as errors may be misguided—like many things, good or bad is seldom black and white. It is a net effect and a matter of context, and an informed strategy should take such considerations into account. The final chapter discusses what we have learned about how to mitigate or suppress these cognitive effects, if and when it is prudent to do so.

PART 1

THE PROBLEM OF MISPERCEPTION

CHAPTER 1

THE FRACTION PROBLEM

In 1979, James Dallas Egbert III, a native of Ohio, was a student at Michigan State University (MSU). Egbert, who went by the name of "Dallas," was a child prodigy, entering MSU at the precocious age of 16.[1] He was also an enthusiastic player of Dungeons and Dragons (D&D), some might say a fanatic. On August 15 of that year, he disappeared. A handwritten message was found in his dorm room that seemed like a suicide note, but no body was found, and an investigation was launched into what befell him.[2]

D&D was a widely popular role-playing game in which players engaged in a joint imaginative exercise and acted out the personas of medieval adventurers in a monster-ridden world full of magic, mystery, and combat. I describe this from personal experience, and with no small sense of nostalgia. In my youth, I was an avid D&D player, entirely engrossed in the game. Like any new trend that engulfs a generation of kids, D&D was strange and unfamiliar to their parents. It was a mysterious black box, full of violence, demons and devils, and sinister magic. In my mother's generation, one had to fear Elvis Presley's gyrating hips; for my generation, parents were suspicious of D&D and kept a careful eye on this odd new fad.

Investigators who were trying to find Dallas learned that he frequently played a form of D&D that involved real life role-playing in the eight miles of labyrinthian steam tunnels that lay beneath MSU. Perhaps something had gone tragically wrong in the tunnels. The media quickly latched onto the D&D angle. Newspaper headlines were nothing less than sensational:[3]

"Missing Youth Could Be on Adventure Game"

"Is Missing Student Victim of Game?"

"Intellectual Fantasy Results in Bizarre Disappearance"

"Student May Have Lost His Life to Intellectual Fantasy Game"

"Student Feared Dead in 'Dungeon' "

An exhaustive search of the steam tunnels turned up a great many curiosities, but nothing that gave a clue as to what happened to Dallas.[4] Ultimately, James Dallas Egbert was recovered alive and in relatively good physical health, on September 12, 1979, almost a full month after his disappearance. How did the detectives finally track him down? They didn't. Dallas called one of the detectives who was looking for him and asked to be retrieved. He was in Morgan City, Louisiana, 1,156 miles away from East Lansing, working in an oil field and living in a dilapidated apartment with some other people, whom he refused to let be identified.[5]

The James Dallas Egbert case focused nationwide attention on D&D. Shockingly, a string of suicides and homicides occurred in the early 1980s, committed by adolescents who frequently played D&D. By 1985, worries about D&D as a game that could cause psychosis, murder, and suicide had developed into a fully matured movement. There was nothing inappropriate about the concern regarding the possible association of playing D&D and suicide. Some correlations are real and may even be causal. If something is potentially dangerous, it should not be ignored, and significant evidence suggested that D&D might truly be dangerous.

Great media attention focused on the concerns that playing D&D was dangerous. Even *60 Minutes* (among the most famous and accomplished U.S. news shows) ran a focused segment on the problem. Gary Gygax (one of two originators of D&D) gave an interview on the show and was asked a direct question: "If you found 12 kids in murder suicide with one connecting factor in each of them, wouldn't you question it?" Gygax answered, "I would certainly do it in a scientific manner, and this is as unscientific as you can get." The segment made the following statement: "There are those who are fearful that the game, in the hands of vulnerable kids, could do harm; and there is evidence that seems to support that view," followed by a list of individuals who played D&D, their ages, and what had happened to them.

So how should one assess the damning evidence put forth? A more detailed analysis subsequently established that 28 teenagers who often played D&D had committed murder, suicide, or both. One might ask, should we just ban the game? What are we waiting for?[6] After all, 28 lives have been lost. What additional facts does one need? Actually, several additional facts are needed.

The first fact is that D&D had become so wildly popular by 1984 that an estimated three million teenagers played it. The second fact is that the general rate of suicides among all U.S. teenagers, at that time, was roughly 120 suicides per year for every one million teenagers. This means that for the three million teenagers who played D&D, one would predict an average annual suicide rate of 360, in the absence of any additional risk factors. In other words, the seemingly striking number of 28 over several years was actually 12-fold lower than the number of suicides one would expect (in the population who played D&D) in a normal year, each and every year. It thus appears that D&D may have been, if anything, therapeutic and decreased the rate of suicides.[7] After considering the number of teenagers playing D&D and the background rate of suicide, the evidence that *60 Minutes* said "seems to support this view" that D&D was dangerous actually supported the opposite view.

A large number of studies has been published in scientific journals, nonscientific journals, the lay press, dissertations, and online writing on this topic (all told more than 150 works).[8] At the end of the day, no credible evidence whatsoever supports the assertion that role-playing games in general, or D&D in particular, increase any risk of dangerous behaviors, including homicide or suicide.[9]

Sadly, almost a year after he returned home, on August 11, 1980, James Dallas Egbert shot a .25-caliber bullet into his head. His life-support machines were turned off six days later.[10] We will never know for sure why Dallas killed himself. But we do know that a credible association between playing D&D and suicide cannot be made and we have no reason to suspect fantasy role-playing games hurt Dallas in any way. It is more likely that D&D actually helped him cope with his struggles. Mental illness and depression do not need an external cause to manifest in the human mind. If a cause must be posited, it is much more likely that it was associated with the societal shaming Dallas seemed to have experienced as a result of being nonheterosexual. Unlike playing D&D, such shaming is well known to actually correlate with an increased risk of suicide.[11]

Given this explanation, the error in misinterpretation is probably pretty clear. But how can we formally describe it? If we can identify a general form of the error that was made, we can remember that form, and be on the lookout for it in other situations. One such instrument to describe this form is the concept of a fraction.

Using the Form of a Fraction as a Conceptual Framework

For many of you, terms like "numerator" and "denominator" may resurrect long-buried memories of the tyranny of a middle-school mathematics teacher or the regrettable trauma of muddling through long story problems trying to figure out percentages. Problems like this:

> Johnny bought $6.00 of fruit and Sally bought $9.00 of fruit. Johnny only bought apples (which were $2.00 apiece) and Sally only bought oranges (which were $1.00 apiece). What percent of the pieces of fruit were apples?[12]

Don't panic. You are likely no longer judged on such abilities, and the rest of this book makes no further mention of story problems. The use of simple mathematical concepts is all we need.

In the definition of a fraction that we will work with, the number on the top is the numerator, which tells you how many of a thing have a certain property. The number on the bottom is the denominator, which tells you how many total things there are.[13] Consider a simple fraction like 1/2, which is just the mathematical representation of the common notion "one-half." In this case, the numerator is the top of the fraction, "1," and the denominator is the bottom of the fraction, "2" (figure 1.1). We can see that a fraction indicates how many of a total population (the denominator) has a particular property (the numerator).

If 1,000 scratch-off lottery tickets are on display in a gas station, then the fraction of winning tickets is the number of winning tickets (i.e., the numerator) over the total number of tickets (i.e., the denominator), or 250/1,000—in other words, 1/4 (i.e., one out of every four, or one-quarter). Importantly, the denominator includes the numerator. In other words, the numerator is just the 250 winning tickets, whereas the denominator is the 250 winning tickets and the 750 losing tickets, to include all 1,000 tickets (figure 1.2).[14]

Many common concepts that humans consider and discuss every day, such as rates, frequencies, percentages, probabilities, risks, and odds, can be expressed using fractions. I am talking about these terms as they are commonly used in English, and not their precise mathematical definitions, which have some subtle (but important) differences. We are concerned with the common use of the words and the concepts to which they are attached.[15]

$$\text{Numerator} \longrightarrow \frac{1}{2} \longleftarrow \text{Denominator}$$

1.1 The simple fraction 1/2.

$$\text{Numerator} \longrightarrow \frac{\overset{\text{Winning}}{250}}{\underset{\text{Winning} \quad \text{Losing}}{250+750}} \longleftarrow \text{Denominator} = \frac{250}{1,000} = 25\%$$

1.2 An example of the numerator and denominator, using lottery tickets.

For example, the common saying that an event is "one in a million," although often not used literally, nevertheless can be captured in mathematical language by the fraction 1/1,000,000. When the *New York Times* reports that "One in seven people in the United States is expected to develop a substance use disorder at some point,"[16] it is the same as saying that substance use disorders occur at a rate of one out of seven people, with a frequency of 1/7, and that 14.3 percent of people will have a substance use problem, that there is a probability of 0.14, and that the risk is 1 in 7 or the odds are 1 to 7.[17] Thus, many common terms and concepts we use in everyday life can be represented in the form of a fraction.

Fractions have particular properties. The numerical value of a fraction can go up or down according to different mechanisms (figure 1.3). An increase in the numerator or a decrease in the denominator both make the value of a fraction go up—one can increase the odds of getting a winning lottery ticket from a display case, to the same extent, by either adding more winning tickets or removing some losing tickets. If we start with 250/1,000 winning tickets, then 25 percent of the tickets are winning (1 in 4 odds or probability of 0.25). If we add 500 winning tickets, the fraction is now 750/1,500, or 50 percent of tickets are winning (1 in 2 odds or probability of 0.50). Alternatively, starting with 250/1,000 tickets, we can subtract 500 losing tickets. The fraction is now

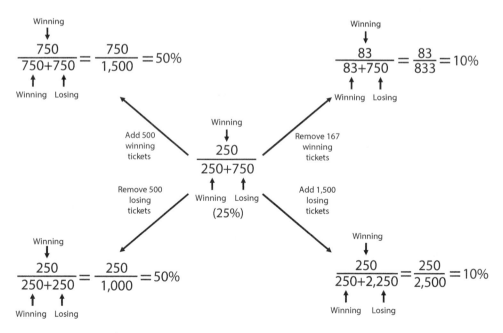

1.3 The odds of getting a winning lottery ticket as affected by different changes to the numerator and denominator.

250/500, or 50 percent of tickets are winning (1 in 2 odds or probability of 0.50). Both approaches increase the value of the fraction by same amount.

Conversely, a decrease in the numerator or an increase in the denominator both make the value of a fraction go down—one can decrease the odds of getting a winning ticket from a display case by removing winning tickets or by adding more losing tickets. If we start with 250/1,000 winning tickets, then 25 percent of the tickets are winning (1 in 4 odds or probability of 0.25). If we take away 167 winning tickets, then the fraction goes down to 83/833 and 10 percent of the tickets are winning (1 in 10 odds or probability of 0.10). Alternatively, we can leave the number of winning tickets the same (250) but add 1,500 losing tickets. Then, the fraction goes down to 250/2,500, or 10 percent of the tickets are winning (1 in 10 odds or probability of 0.10).

The depth to which the simple properties of fractions are intuitively misunderstood by people runs deep. A fairly humorous, albeit embarrassing example of this was discovered in the 1980s with regards to a great American standard— the fast-food hamburger. McDonald's quarter-pounder (i.e., 1/4 pounder) had been a dominant force in the hamburger market since it was introduced in 1971. In an effort to knock the 1/4 pounder off its pedestal, A&W introduced a burger that was favored by consumers in blinded taste tests and cost less than the 1/4 pounder. Even better, the A&W burger was a larger quantity of meat, coming in at one-third of a pound (1/3 pound). Sadly, for A&W, their new 1/3-pound hamburger was a flop. Once it was clear that it was failing despite its many virtues, analysis of customer focus groups demonstrated why people were not purchasing it. Consumers thought 1/3 pound of meat was less than 1/4 pound, because 3 is less than 4.[18]

Common language we use to describe changes in fractions can also lead to counterintuitive results. For instance, consider if a stock has a value of $1,000/ share. Then say that its value goes down by 50 percent but later goes up by 50 percent. To many people, it seems that the stock should now be valued at $1,000/share, after all, it went down and then up again by the same amount. Actually, it did not. Instead, it went down and then up by the same percentage. When it went down by 50 percent, the value was $500/share. When it then went up by 50 percent, the value was now $750/share. The percentage change is a function of the value that is changing.

Alternatively, consider the meaning of the percentage increase in the number of people afflicted by certain diseases. According to the Centers for Disease Control and Prevention (CDC), there are (on average) seven cases of plague each year in the United States.[19] In contrast, more than 800,000 people die from vascular disease in the United States each year (e.g., heart attack or stroke). So, someone might tell you that the number of plague cases and deaths from vascular disease both increased by 300 percent. In the case of plague that would equate to only twenty-one more cases, but in the case of vascular disease, it would equate to 2.4 million more deaths. Even though both values went up by 300 percent, the numerical magnitude of the change between the two diseases is not even close.

Ignoring the Denominator

How can we utilize the concept of a fraction to formally explain what happened in the case of teenage suicides and playing D&D? The likelihood of someone who plays D&D committing murder or suicide is a simple fraction. Those who both play D&D and also commit murder or suicide are on the top of the fraction (numerator) and the total number of people who play D&D are on the bottom (denominator). The fraction would appear like this:

People who play D&D and commit murder or suicide / Everyone who plays D&D

The media and those concerned were focusing on the numerator but did not take the denominator into account.

Why is ignoring the denominator such a problem? If I focus on only the numerator and don't consider the denominator, then each of the statements shown in figure 1.4 seem to be correct. When considering the effect of the denominator, however, each of these statements is clearly wrong. Calculation of risk takes the form of a fraction, and as such, unless one accurately considers

$$\frac{1}{2} \quad \text{is less than} \quad \frac{5}{1,000} \quad \text{because 1 is less than 5}$$

$$\frac{5}{1,000} \quad \text{is greater than} \quad \frac{1}{2} \quad \text{because 5 is greater than 1}$$

$$\frac{1}{1,000,000} \quad \text{is the same as} \quad \frac{1}{20} \quad \text{because } 1 = 1$$

1.4 Clearly incorrect statements that appear to be true if the denominator is ignored.

both the top and bottom of the fraction, then one cannot determine the risk. Yet, when faced with a number of events (in this case, children who played D&D and committed murder or suicide, the numerator), people often jump to a risk assessment without considering the total number (in this case, the number of kids playing D&D, the denominator).[20]

Focusing on the numerator alone is not always an error; sometimes, the denominator is not relevant, and its inclusion could lead to an incorrect result. Sometimes, we simply need to know a numerical value and are not concerned about the rate, frequency, percentage, probability, risk, or odds. For example, I might be a healthcare provider who is trying to adequately stock my pharmacy with medication for heart disease. What I really need to know is how many people in my community have heart disease. For these purposes, it is irrelevant to me what *percentage* of the population has heart disease. I have no particular need of the denominator (the total number of people in my community). I only need to know the numerator (the absolute number of people with heart disease regardless of how many people are in the community).

Whenever an issue of rate, frequency, percentage, probability, risk, or odds is important, then both the numerator and denominator are needed. To focus on one to the exclusion of the other can lead to error. An epidemiologist who was trying to figure out the rates of heart disease between two different cities could make little use of the numerator alone. Knowing that there were 10,000 cases last year in each city is not useful without knowing how many people live in each city.[21] With just the numerator (10,000), it looks like the rate of heart disease between cities might be the same—after all, both had the same number of cases. This determination changes drastically, however, if one learns that the first city is a booming metropolis like New York (with approximately eight million inhabitants), whereas the second city is a small Midwestern town with twenty thousand inhabitants.[22] When assessing frequency or risk, neither the numerator nor the denominator alone is sufficient; both are needed for either one to be meaningful.

None of this is profound. Humans intuitively recognize instances like these. If someone said to you that the risk of heart disease is the same in the large city and the small Midwestern town because they have the name number of cases, it would be pretty clear that the statement is confusing risk of disease with number of people afflicted. In many cases, however, human cognition does not make the leap to ask what the size of the denominator is or even to consider that there is one. This tendency is often subconscious, and people remain unaware that they are not taking the whole fraction into account.

Regrettably, publication of data-driven analysis is not compelling to many people, who prefer their intuitive interpretations of the world. Part of this may be intrigue. In the artful words of Jon Peterson with regards to the D&D issue, "The myth of the game that drove college kids insane was simply more powerful than the dull reality that so much hype and furor derived from a private investigator's misguided hunch."[23] However, it seems to go much deeper than that. Humans have the persistent tendency to notice only numerators. Recently, the *New York Times* wrote a follow-up piece about the panic surrounding D&D in historical terms.[24] As the article points out, the error is consistent, ongoing, and in no way restricted to D&D: "Today, parental anxieties have turned to videos, notably those dripping with gore. Can it be mere coincidence, some ask, that the mass killers in Colorado at Columbine High School and the Aurora movie theater, and at the grade school in Newtown Conn., all played violent electronic games?"

The shootings at Columbine High School, Sandy Hook Elementary School, and the seemingly endless stream of mass shootings, before and since, are horrific events of profound tragedy. We should be vigilant in seeking causes of violent behavior and doing everything we can to prevent them. The important (and tragic) point is that seeking such causes cannot stop with finding a few things the assailants had in common and then trying to ban these things without more detailed analysis that includes the whole picture (i.e., the denominator). In other words, like the D&D case, is the rate of violent acts among adolescents playing violent electronic games higher than it is in all adolescents in general? If so, is it a causal factor?[25] As is good and appropriate, research into this issue is ongoing.

Indeed, an association between violent video games and aggressive behavior has been reported in multiple studies,[26] even though this association may be due to what is called publication bias (a particular manifestation of the type of error we are exploring in this book that is discussed in detail in chapter 10).[27] Thankfully, scientists continue to study this question using methods that control for such confounders. Failing to assess the denominator not only risks our focusing energy on the vilification of benign, or even beneficial things, but also distracts and misdirects our attention from what the real causal problems may be.

Ignoring the Denominator Is Widespread in Political Dialogue

Politicians frequently ignore or purposely obscure the denominator to manipulate political facts. Consider a common type of claim made by politicians and political parties, pretty much every economic quarter and each electoral cycle. Claims like "we made the biggest tax cut in history," or "we created more jobs than anyone in history," or "we had the largest economic growth in history," or "under my opponent, the economy lost more value than in any recession in the history of the country." The arguments would not be made, and repeated over and over, if they weren't convincing. But many times, these claims are simply pointing to the dollar amount or the number of jobs without considering the size of the economy or work force, that is, they focus on the numerator and ignore the denominator.

Consider that if today the Dow Jones drops by 182 points, it is a slightly down day, but it is really no big deal. The famous stock market crash of 1929, however, was a drop of this amount and it was disastrous. The Dow Jones at its peak was around 381 in the year 1929 before the crash, whereas it was over 30,000 in the year 2021. So, a $182 drop in 1929 was a loss of 48 percent; the same drop in 2021 is less than 1 percent. It would be correct to say that the stock market had larger decreases under presidents Carter, Reagan, Bush, Clinton, Bush, Obama, and Trump than it ever did under Herbert Hoover as our country slid into the Great Depression if, that is, you consider just the numerator (the dollar change in the market) and not the denominator (the value of the market).

Consider the U.S. Presidential campaign of 2016. Then-candidate Donald Trump repeatedly argued that we need to close our borders to immigrants and aggressively deport undocumented immigrants. The argument put forth by Donald Trump was the need to protect citizens from criminal acts by immigrants. He repeatedly referred to the murder of a U.S. citizen named Kathryn Steinle by an undocumented immigrant named Juan Francisco López-Sánchez. The argument was simple. Kathryn Steinle was killed by an undocumented immigrant; therefore, undocumented immigrants are dangerous. So, getting rid of undocumented immigrants will remove dangerous people and thus protect citizens by decreasing murder.

Implicit in Donald Trump's rhetoric is the idea that immigrants are more dangerous than U.S. citizens. This is easy to infer, given Trump's own words: "When Mexico sends its people, they're not sending their best . . . They're bringing drugs. They're bringing crime. They're rapists. And some, I assume, are good people."[28]

Certainly, if Mexico actually were selectively sending criminals to the United States, then this would be a serious concern. To properly understand the situation, however, we need more information. We have to know the top of the fraction (i.e., how many murders are carried out by immigrants each year, the numerator) as well as the bottom of the fraction (i.e., how many total immigrants are in the United States, the denominator). Then, to assess relative risk, we must compare this to another fraction (i.e., the same fraction applied to nonimmigrants), in particular, the following: number of murders carried out by nonimmigrant citizens/number of total nonimmigrant citizens. The outcome of this analysis is really quite clear.

Numerous studies have shown that crime rates among immigrants occur at a much lower frequency than nonimmigrants.[29] In other words, after taking both the numerators and the denominators into account, citizens born in the United States are more likely to commit violent crimes than immigrants are. The same finding holds true even if one focuses solely on undocumented immigrants.[30]

If this is correct, we would have a lower rate of crime (often called per capita crime) with more immigrants. Indeed, as immigration increased in the 1990s, the United States experienced a steady decline in per capita crime during that decade. Of course, we cannot distinguish between simple correlation and causation, but we cannot ignore the data either. The data are what the data are, and they certainly show what we could expect if immigrants are less dangerous than natural-born citizens. The observed decrease in crime along with increased immigration is so significant that it is relatively immune to statistical manipulation. As Alex Nowrasteh, an analyst at the Cato Institute, explains, "There's no way I can mess with the numbers to get a different conclusion."[31]

Of course, we could be concerned that this argument has altered the fraction along the way. Although much anti-immigration rhetoric speaks against immigration in general, Trump's claims seemed to be focused on immigrants from Mexico. Perhaps immigrants from Mexico really are more likely to be criminals, but immigrants from other parts of the world are so law abiding that they offset the effects. This is not the case, however, and the same trends are observed when one limits analysis to immigrants from Mexico alone.[32] Notably, subsequent to the presidential election of 2016, Juan Francisco López-Sánchez was tried and acquitted of all murder and manslaughter charges by a jury who found that the shooting was an unintentional and horrible accident. Juan Francisco López-Sánchez *was* convicted of having a firearm as a felon.

The claim is not that immigrants do not commit crimes. Clearly, many crimes are carried out by individuals who have immigrated to the United States. However, it does not follow that because some immigrants carry out crimes, therefore crimes are more likely to be carried out by immigrants. To justify this conclusion, we would need to observe a greater *rate* of crime by immigrants compared with crimes by nonimmigrants, and this is simply not the case. Many politicians do not make this comparison, however, either because they do not know that they should or because taking such factors into account does not support their agenda. Clearly, Ms. Steinle's murder was a horrible thing. But the greatest way to pay respect to Ms. Steinle would come from strategies that target the actual causes of violent crime.

Changing the Outcome by Kicking Out Data

In 1574, in the Scottish Village of Loch Ficseanail, a man named Duncan MacLeod was drinking with his close friend Hamish. Duncan made the following claim to Hamish: "All true Scotsmen can hold their liquor without fail!" About this time, a tall handsome man with a red beard and a plaid kilt walked into the bar and ordered a glass of scotch. By the time he had finished his drink, he was slurring his speech, seemed disoriented, and proceeded to fall off his barstool onto the ground, where he lay unconscious. Hamish looked at Duncan curiously.

"Well," Hamish said, "I guess you were wrong when you claimed that all true Scotsmen can hold their liquor."

"I was not wrong," bellowed Duncan, "for you see, this fellow lying on the floor is clearly no true Scotsman."

This is a version of the classic story that gives rise to the no true Scotsman fallacy. The initial claim made by Duncan is no less a fraction or percentage than the earlier examples. Basically, it is saying that 100 percent of True Scotsmen can hold their liquor. One can guarantee that the statement is always true by selectively kicking Scotsmen who can't hold their liquor out of the fraction (i.e., removing them from the club of true Scotsmen). This story is crafted to make the fallacy clear, and it is easy to dismiss this as a quaint tale that makes a good joke.

In the real world, people engage in this kind of thinking all the time. Sometimes it is obvious, such as Donald Trump's statement during the 2016 election: "I will totally accept the results of this great and historic presidential election— if I win."[33] In other words, the only election that is a legitimate election is an election I win; therefore, I will win 100 percent of legitimate elections. Indeed, President Trump really was dedicated to this notion, accounting for his relentless efforts to challenge the legitimacy of the 2020 election. In his view, the strongest evidence that the election must have been rigged is the outcome. Trump did not win, so therefore it is not a legitimate election (if a True Scotsman can't hold their liquor, then they aren't a True Scotsman). Although clear in this case, the same type of error often manifests in subtler ways.

We constantly hear about the unemployment rate in America—it is one of the key economic indicators that is used to assess the health of our economy. Because this is a rate, it therefore fits the form of a fraction. At first glance this does not seem to be complicated: the unemployment rate should be a fraction with the number of people who don't have jobs on the top (numerator) and the total number of people on the bottom (denominator). But the fraction cannot actually include all people who don't have jobs, because that would include children too young to work, people unable to work (due to disability or illness), and people who do not want to work (e.g., retired people or those who choose not to seek employment). The unemployment rate would be immense, and the figure would not be meaningful. This is the opposite of the no-true-Scotsman fallacy, as individuals who do not qualify for the fraction are being included erroneously. It would be like bragging that the rate of prostate cancer in America could never rise to more than 50 percent if you include all Americans in your calculations (i.e., both people who were born with prostates and those who weren't).

The real issue here is what constitutes an unemployed person? The standard definition of an unemployed person is someone who does not have a job, is able to work, and is looking for employment (i.e., has applied for a job in the past four weeks). This means that people who want a job and are seeking one (but not in the past four weeks) are neither employed nor unemployed—they are kicked out of the fraction just like the drunken Scotsman. People who have stopped seeking employment are not counted at all. This means that if the job market gets bad enough that people who want to work grow discouraged and stop applying for a few weeks, then the unemployment rate will drop even though the number of employed people has not changed. The point is that an economy that is adding many new jobs and an economy in which jobs are so hard to find that people seeking work give up for a few weeks both result in a drop in unemployment rates.

When we are given a term like unemployment rate, we are provided with a single number, like 8 percent. Understanding the fraction behind this number and knowing how the numerator and denominator are defined is essential to interpreting the single numbers we are given (e.g., unemployment rate). Regrettably, politicians and others with particular agendas purposefully exploit this type of fraction to manipulate opinion and promote misunderstanding that favors their priorities. We seldom are given the specific particulars of fractions (such as unemployment rate), which remain invisible to us unless we seek them out. We are given only the single number that comes out of the calculation.

The Special Case of Averages

On May 8, 2020, as the shutdown in response to COVID-19 was making its effect felt on the economy, the U.S. Labor Department reported an amazingly strong growth in wages.[34] Did companies suddenly realize how much they valued their workers and how tough times were and thus increase wages? No, actually, wages didn't change at all—at least not for most individuals. Government statistics are often an average that is given to assess how a group of people is performing. The average is calculated by adding the values of each member of a group and then dividing by the number of people in the group. This is a type of fraction. An important distinction adds special properties to an average not found in the other fractions we have discussed thus far. An average is not a fraction in which we are counting the number of things with a certain property (in the numerator) over the total number of things (in the denominator). Rather, the numerator is the sum of quantitative values attributed to each thing, such as income. Consider the following:

Three people each earned a salary. The three salaries were 2, 4, and 6. What is the average salary?

$$(2 + 4 + 6)/3 = 4$$

Note that there are different ways to get to the same average. For example, if all three people made a salary of 4, then the average also would be 4:

$$(4 + 4 + 4)/3 = 4$$

Or if the salaries were 1, 1, and 10, the average would likewise be 4.

$$(1 + 1 + 10)/3 = 4$$

So, although the average is an important measure, it does not tell you anything about how the numbers are distributed. This is where the field of statistics steps in to consider the properties of the population under analysis.

How does an understanding of averages help us make sense of the U.S. Labor Department report? Because calculations of average salary apply only to those who actually are making a salary, people who lost their jobs are removed from the calculation (in other words, they are kicked out of the fraction). Job loss was highest among those making the least, so the average salaries (of those remaining) was higher, but not because anyone's wage had gone up. Instead, lower wage earners were removed from the fraction. As reported by the *Washington Post*, "So, nobody's actually earning more. It's just that many of the lowest earners are now earning nothing."[35]

Not appreciating all of the properties of the fraction behind a number, and the rules by which it is modified, leads to claims, perceptions, and beliefs that do not reflect reality. This is the power of fractions to deceive.

Talking Past Each Other Using Different Fractions

On Tuesday, July 28, 2020, Donald Trump was interviewed by journalist Jonathan Swan on the HBO show *Axios*. The interview caused quite an uproar, with opponents of Trump claiming it pointed to his incompetence.[36] The specific exchange that caught everyone's attention was an argument on whether the United States was doing better or worse than other countries in its response to the COVID-19 pandemic. Listening carefully to the discussion, it becomes clear that President Trump and Jonathan Swan were really arguing about which fraction should be used to figure out what was actually happening with the pandemic.

President Trump acknowledged that the United States had more cases than any other country in the world, but he claimed that this was misleading, because the United States also was testing many more people; hence, of course, more cases would be identified. President Trump was absolutely correct in this regard. It is true that if two countries each had the same rate of infection (cases/number of people) and one country tested 10 times more people than the other country, then the country that tested more would detect 10 times more cases.

This analysis, however, focuses on the numerator and ignores the denominator. Instead, if we divide the number of cases by the number of people tested, then the two countries would have identical rates of infection.[37] This is the power of fractions: they allow interpretation of what the number of cases really mean in the context of the population. So, in this regard, Trump could have been absolutely correct when he stated that "[b]ecause we are so much better at testing than any other country in the world, we show more cases."

Although more testing will lead to reporting a greater number of cases, this does not mean that reporting a greater number of cases can only be due to more testing. Many different things can lead to more cases, including an increased rate of infection. We can easily determine the actual cause of increased numbers of cases with the use of the right fraction. If Trump's claim was correct, then the fraction (positive tests/total number people tested) should not be higher in the United States than elsewhere. Regrettably for the United States, this was not the case. On July 27, 2020, the day before the *Axios* interview, the United States had the third highest percentage of positive tests of nations being monitored, with an 8.4 percent positivity rate compared with countries doing much better, including the United Kingdom (0.5 percent) and South Korea (0.7 percent).[38] In light of this fact, to say that the United States had more cases only because it was testing more people is not supportable. Regrettably, Trump's claims do not hold up to the available data and are a distortion of the truth.

To be fair, however, there are many ways to define the numerator and denominator of a fraction that can alter its properties. Countries might be using different testing methodologies that have a range of sensitivities and specificities for the virus, which would alter the numerator. Regarding the denominator, two countries could have identical rates of infection with one country performing tests only on people who have symptoms and the other country broadly testing asymptomatic people who have had contact with infected people, or even as part of random testing. In other words, the actual fraction being measured in country 1 is (positive tests/sick people tested) and in country 2 it is (positive tests/sick and nonsick people tested). Country 1 would report a higher rate of infection than country 2 (even if the overall rate of infection was identical). Because country 1 is selecting the population that is being tested (using symptoms as a screening tool), the incidence of positive tests will be higher. This is a case of a faulty comparison in which it appears the formula for fractions are the same, but they actually are different. It's an easy mistake to make. The label "positive test rate" describes both fractions, even though the fractions are fundamentally different based on who is included in the fraction.

This same problem can occur within a single nation over time. For example, early in the pandemic resources for testing were limited, and only sick people were being tested. Later, as testing resources became more widespread, contacts and random people were also being tested. Thus, the frequency of positive cases would drop, making it look as though the epidemic was getting better even though it wasn't. This could produce such a large drop as to make it look like the epidemic was improving even while the epidemic was worsening.

To avoid these types of errors, Jonathan Swan focused not on the number of positive tests that were being reported, but rather the death rate (number of deaths from COVID-19/total population of the country). Why would this make a difference? First, there is no ambiguity in the numerator—dead is dead (although one could argue about the actual cause of death, and some people did). Second, the denominator is the total population of the country, which is a fixed value. Jonathan Swan informed Trump how poorly the United States was doing in the number of deaths per total population compared with other nations and explained how this figure was increasing in the United States. If Trump was correct that increases in reported cases did not reflect higher rates of infection, but were only due to more testing (i.e., the epidemic wasn't getting worse), then deaths would not increase.

> *Jonathan Swan*: "The figure I look at is Death, and death is going up now . . . it's 1,000 cases per day."[39]
> *Trump*: "Take a look at some of these charts . . . we're gonna look . . . Right here, the United States is lowest in numerous categories, we're lower than the world, we're lower than Europe. . . . right here, here's Case Death."
> *Swan*: "Oh you're doing death as a proportion of cases I'm talking about death as a proportion of population; that's where the U.S. is really bad, much worse than South Korea, Germany, etc."
> *Trump*: "You can't do that; you have to go by the cases."

In this instance, both Trump and Swan were saying correct things. Trump was correct that compared with other countries, the United States had a low number (death/diagnosed case of COVID-19) and Swan was also correct that the United States had a high number (death from COVID-19/population). Trump was using one fraction, and Swan was using another. They disagreed on which was the correct fraction to use as well as what the respective fractions indicated. Swan's fraction indicated that if you lived in the United States you were more likely to die from COVID-19 than if you lived in another country. In contrast, Trump's fraction indicated that once you were diagnosed with COVID-19 in the United States, you were less likely to die than in other countries. Trump's fraction was important regarding issues of quality of patient care but had no relevance to how many people were getting infected or how well the United States was handling public health measures to limit the spread of COVID-19.

It is unclear if Trump really believed that his fraction was the correct analysis or if he understood it all too well and was just grasping at straws to find any metric where the United States was doing better than other nations. It seems clear, however, that his conclusions were simply incorrect, and not only because of the previous arguments. The actual number of people who die from COVID-19 is what it is, regardless of whether or not we detect infection. Our testing affects if we count a death as being caused by COVID-19, but in and of itself, it does not change whether the person dies. As such, it is meaningful to consider that the overall number of Americans that died in 2020 was considerably higher than what was predicted based upon annual averages (since 2013), and the timing of increased deaths lined up with the timing of COVID-19 infections.[40] If it looks like we have more deaths only because we are doing more testing, then why did the absolute number of people dying dramatically increase?

Maneuvers to adjust fractions or use the incorrect fractions to argue an agenda-driven point are by no means particular to Trump. This is common among politicians of any party. Although this example focuses on the United States, because the narrative is so clear, politicians in essentially all nations utilize such ploys, from autocratic monarchies to representative republics. That it is common makes it no less misleading or manipulative. This example illustrates how the issue of what fractions you choose, and how you are using them, are baked into the real-time events that unfold in front of us every day. This case also demonstrates why we need a firm concept of fractions, how they work, and what they mean to untwist whether claims are in line with reality.

Fractions Fractions Everywhere nor Any a Chance to Think

Once you develop the habit of looking for fractions, you can start to see them everywhere—and you can start to see where fractions are not being used when they should be. A great example of this is in self-help systems, for both people and corporations. Consider how often you have seen a book or seminar entitled something like "The Five Habits of Self-Made Millionaires" or "Strategies of Highly Successful and Disruptive Startup Companies." Actually, the list seems like an endless conveyor belt of the same types of claims, over and over again, ad nauseam. The statement "The Five Habits of Self-Made Millionaires" implies that doing these five things contributed to the ability of others to make lots of money, *and* if you do the same five things, you likely will have the same success. This sounds reasonable. Something is tragically missing, however. You guessed it: we are ignoring a vital component of the fraction at play.

In any given system for success, from personal habits to corporate culture, let's just grant that the success stories are real and were caused by some strategy (i.e., not just dumb luck). The analysis cannot simply consist of noticing the characteristics of the people or corporations and emulating them. Why not? It would be an inevitably true statement that the following are traits of the richest 10 people in the United States: (1) breathing, (2) eating, (3) blinking, (4) urinating, (5) defecating, and (6) yawning.[41] The characteristics that are usually described in the self-help programs we are discussing are more reasonably associated with success than are breathing and eating, but that does not resolve the issue we are discussing. The issue is not what characteristics are found in successful people; the issue is what characteristics are found in successful people *and not* in less successful people. If an activity increases the likelihood of success, then it should be present at a higher rate in successful people and corporations. When you are seeking a rate, then what you are considering is in the form of a fraction.

The next time you encounter a success system like we are describing, see whether there is an assessment of how often the habits or traits being described are present in people or corporations who are not successful, or even in those who are clearly failures. If you are attending a seminar on this system, ask the question: "where is the data on how frequently these traits are found in the general population and is it higher or lower than highly successful people?" Even better, do not accept a single anecdotal example as the evidence, but rather ask for the data on groups of people. In my experience, you won't get a good answer, if you get an answer at all. (Sadly, you won't get your money back either, even if you ask very nicely.) In most cases, the real secret to success is coming up with a system that promises to teach the secrets of success and then selling books and running seminars.

Summary

In this chapter, I introduced fractions and showed how their properties affect descriptions of real-life situations and interpretations of claims of fact. These examples illustrated how not considering that a fraction is at play, not taking the whole fraction into account, or not using the correct fraction can lead to confusion, miscommunication, and—in some cases—manipulation. Learning to recognize when fractions are at play is essential. Fractions are almost inevitably involved when discussing rates, frequencies, percentages, probabilities, averages, risks, and odds.

Once we learn to look for them, fractions are everywhere, although not always obvious on the surface. Having recognized that a fraction is involved, understanding the nature of the fraction and the rules by which the numerator and denominator are defined (and manipulated) is essential to understanding what the information really means. Learning to identify the nuances of how fractions are defined and manipulated to generate claims of fact can change the way we understand the world.

Most of the examples in this chapter have focused on circumstances external to ourselves. Applying the concept of a fraction is not limited to the external world, but rather it extends to understanding what happens inside our minds. This will be the focus of the next chapter.

CHAPTER 2

HOW OUR MINDS FRACTIONATE
THE WORLD

Humans tend to perceive a rich and complex world all around them. Our minds, however, distort the frequency of the things we encounter, not only by what we can sense but also by what we notice and remember. Our intuitions of the frequency of things are often a far cry from what occurs in the external world. We do not need other's manipulation for this to happen, we do it to ourselves, as a fundamental property of human perception and cognition—and worst of all, we are often entirely unaware that we do it.[1]

The Filter of Our Sensory Organs

Our range of hearing is from 20 Hz to 20 kHz. The world is full of sound waves outside this range, but we are not capable of hearing them. Our eyes can see light in the range of 380 to 740 nanometers, but we are oblivious to infrared or ultraviolet light outside this range. Microscopes reveal a world of details, creatures, and object too small for our unaided eyes to see. Our olfaction and taste can detect the presence of certain chemical entities, while having no ability whatsoever to detect others. Our tactile system can detect wrinkles down to 10 nanometers in length, but no smaller. Smaller wrinkles are there, but to human fingers, they feel seamless and smooth. The world is full of sounds and light and chemicals and textures that fall outside our perceptual limits. They are not available to us, and as a result, they do not affect how we experience the world.

What about the information that our senses can detect: How much of it do we notice? People often are surprised to learn how oblivious we are to much of the input coming into our senses. We sample miniscule bits of the available information and infer the rest of the world, even though it is right in front of us and all around us.[2] One example is found in a fascinating body of work about how people read. In 1975, George W. McConkie and Keith Rayner attempted to ask a seemingly simple question:[3] How much can a person read within one visual gaze—that is, within a "single fixation"? To answer this question, McConkie and Rayner devised a rather ingenious experiment.

They built an apparatus and programmed a computer such that it could detect where a person was looking on a computer screen of text. The computer's memory was programmed to contain a coherent page of readable text. The computer, however, created a window around the portion of text the person was looking at and displayed the actual text only in that window; any text that fell outside that window was changed to gibberish (a mishmash of random letters). This process was entirely unknown to the subject, who believed they simply were reading a page of regular text on a computer. An example of how this looked is shown in figure 2.1.

As the person read the passage of text and their gaze continued to move, the computer shifted the window to keep up with their gaze, changing whatever letters now fell into the window into readable text and reverting the letters that no longer were in the window into garbled text. By varying the size of the

Graphology means personality diagnosis from hand writing.

This was changed to the following line of text:

*

Cnojkaiazp wsore jsnconality diagnosis tnaw kori mnlflrz.

⌞_____⌟

window of non-gibberish

2.1 An example of how a line of text would appear to a subject with a point of fixation on the asterisk.

Source: Reprinted by permission from Springer Nature Customer Service Centre GmbH: George W. McConkie and Keith Rayner, "The Span of Effective Stimulus During a Fixation in Reading," *Perception and Psychophysics* 17, no. 6 (1975), © Psychonomic Society, Inc.

window of readable letters, and determining when the person noticed gibberish, the experimenters could tell how many letters a person was able to perceive within a single fixation. In other words, people would notice the garbled text only when the window of nongibberish was smaller than their window of perception. Through this approach, and with follow-up studies, the researchers determined that people identify a letter of fixation and that the window of perception extends 2–3 characters to the left and 17–18 characters to the right (the letter of fixation is indicated by the asterisk in figure 2.1).[4] The exact nature of the window depends on the size and type of text, the size of the words, and the direction of reading—as some languages are read in different directions.

Although interesting, the size of the reading window is not the point for the current discussion; rather, it is the rest of the text that one is not perceiving when reading 20 characters at a time. What came out of these experiments is the appreciation that when reading, people are not aware of the text outside their narrow window of observation. As explained by Steven Sloman and Philip Fernback in their book *The Knowledge Illusion: Why We Never Think Alone*, the subjects are entirely oblivious to the rest of the document:

> Even if everything outside just a few words is random letters, participants believe they are reading normal text. For anyone standing behind the reader looking at the screen, most of what they see is nonsense, and yet the reader has no idea. Because what the reader is seeing at any given moment is meaningful, the reader assumes everything is meaningful.[5]

For all you know, this page that you are currently reading has the very same properties, and you simply cannot tell just by reading it at a normal distance. It is not that the letters that turn to gibberish, which you do not notice turning to gibberish, are outside of your field of vision, but rather that the light photons reflecting off of those letters are still hitting your eyes, but your focus and perception is such that you do not notice them. The only way you perceive them is if they stay gibberish when you look right at them, as in the case of hglaithceayl—flgoenicisth kkjanreiah.

The issue is not limited to odd laboratory situations of coherent reading windows surrounded by garbled text. Consider your ability to focus on a conversation you are having with a person across the table from you in a crowded restaurant. The words of other diners are still hitting your ears, as are all the sounds of the restaurant, you just don't notice them. Even if you try, you are not able to listen simultaneously to multiple conversations, at least not very well. This is the basis of misdirection in stage magic; what you do not notice happening is not hidden. Rather, the brilliance of the trick is that it is right in front of you, but you do not notice it because your attention is focused on something else. Your inattention to the mechanics of the trick makes you functionally blind to it, so it appears to be magic.[6] This has been called "inattentional blindness," and it is one way human perception filters input from the world around us.

In their book *The Invisible Gorilla: How Our Intuitions Deceive Us*, Christopher Chabris and Daniel Simons provide extensive examples of situations in which we do not perceive the world in front of us.[7] A famous example of this is when subjects are asked to watch a film in which players wearing either white or black jerseys are dribbling several basketballs and passing the balls back and forth between them. The viewers are instructed to count the number of passes of balls from players wearing one color of jersey. Some of those watching get the number of ball passes correct, and others don't, but that is not the point. The point is that 46 percent of people fail to notice the person in a gorilla suit, who walks across the middle of the screen, thumps its chest, and then goes wandering off again.[8] Because the viewers are focusing their attention on counting the passes, they don't notice the rest of the scene; they have inattentional blindness for the gorilla.

Inattentional blindness is not just a quaint trick that can be evoked with movies of basketballs and gorillas. Rather it occurs in much more serious ways in real life, contributing considerably to motorcycle fatalities in what is described as "looked-but-failed-to-see" crashes. This consists of a vehicle (typically a car) cutting off an oncoming motorcycle. Because of inattentional blindness, drivers are much more likely to perceive an oncoming car, than an oncoming motorcycle, even though both are clearly visible, are moving, and the driver is staring directly at them.[9] Because they are looking for cars, cars are all they tend to see—they are oblivious to the rest of the world in front of them, including the motorcycle.

How Our Minds Distort the Fraction of the Things We Do Perceive

I grew up in the northern suburbs of Chicago. Each winter vacation, our family drove down to Florida for a two-week holiday. Years earlier, while in the military, my father had been in a plane that had bad engine troubles in the air, followed by a very precarious landing, which had convinced him that flying was dangerous. So, our family drove everywhere, because it was safer, at least in our estimation. Our main form of amusement in Florida was hanging out at the beach; however, I had a strong aversion to entering the Gulf Waters. The movie world had just been taken by storm by *Jaws*; I was *not* going into the ocean. No, I was going to live a long life and not take any reckless risks, like flying or exposing myself to shark attacks. I am happy to report that my clever strategy and my thoughtful approach to life worked exactly as planned. As of the time of writing this, I have neither been in a plane crash nor have I been attacked by a shark, and by all measures I am still very much alive.

Personal experience, both that you have had yourself and stories you have heard from others (i.e., anecdotal evidence), is important information to consider when making future choices. Avoiding a situation with which you have had a bad personal experience is acting rationally based on available data, albeit a small amount of data. If you have heard stories of people dying while engaging in a certain activity, it seems a good idea to avoid doing it. Watching a news story about how people are being killed in certain situations and then avoiding those situations is just common sense. However, when assessing the relative risks of doing one thing versus another (like driving to Florida versus flying), choosing personal experiences and anecdotal evidence over broad population-based data can be highly problematic. Regrettably, this is precisely what humans tend to do.

As we explored in chapter 1, risk fits the form of a fraction. To properly compare the risk of driving with the risk of flying, my father could have gone to the library and searched for information regarding the risk of dying in a car crash versus a plane crash—today, one could just search on the internet. Of course, many additional levels of detail could be examined to inform probabilistic thinking, such as the airline, the type of plane, the type of car, the route taken, and weather conditions. Our family did not do any of this; in fact, we did not even think to do it—and that is precisely the point. It is a human tendency to navigate issues of risk by simply avoiding things that one hears scary stories about, without considering the actual risks involved.

Cognitive psychologists have made much progress in defining patterns of reasoning that humans are prone to in different situations and under different circumstances. Amos Tversky and Daniel Kahneman were instrumental in developing our understanding of "heuristics." A heuristic is a process by which human minds rapidly solve complex problems by replacing them with analogous but simpler problems. Heuristics have been described as rule-of-thumb thinking or as a "mental shortcut." This process can easily be demonstrated using a famous example of purchasing a baseball and a bat. Consider the following problem described by Daniel Kahneman and Shane Frederick:

> A bat and a ball cost $1.10 in total.
> The bat costs $1.00 more than the ball
> How much does the ball cost?[10]

The majority of people will answer that the ball costs $0.10. That way the bat and the ball cost $1.10 cents together and the problem has been solved.

But wait a minute. If one reflects further on the answer, then they will discover a problem: $1.00 is only $0.90 greater than $0.10. So the bat costing $1.00

and the ball costing $0.10 does not fulfill the condition that the bat costs $1.00 more than the ball. The problem can be fulfilled only by making the bat cost $1.05 and the ball cost $0.05.

This example shows how intuitive thinking arrives at an answer quickly, but in this particular case, the answer is wrong. The mind has substituted a simpler problem (that it can easily solve) for the more complex problem. Moreover, this substitution is subconscious, happening unbeknownst to the person who has made it. Through a process called "attribute substitution," people think they are analyzing the actual problem in front of them, without recognizing that they have subconsciously substituted a simpler problem for the more complex one.

One particular heuristic, the availability heuristic, is relevant to how humans assess the types of problems we have been discussing (i.e., rates, frequencies, percentages, probabilities, risks and odds). In the words of Tversky and Kahneman: "A person is said to employ the availability heuristic whenever he estimates frequency or probability by the ease with which instances or associations can be brought to mind."[11]

Notably, the availability heuristic often works extremely well. The utility of the availability heuristic, however, depends on the assumption that the more easily an association comes to mind, the more likely it actually is to occur. In the words of Tversky, Slovic, and Kahneman, the availability heuristic "uses strength of association as a basis for the judgment of frequency."[12] If we could grant the assumption that your personal experience, or rather your active memory thereof, was an accurate representation of actual frequencies, then the availability heuristic would not be problematic. Sometimes this assumption holds, and in this way, the availability heuristic can offer a distinct advantage. Moreover, favoring personal experience versus broad statistical data may be a better approach when our microenvironment is different from the rest of the world. If you have experienced an earthquake in your home, then you probably live in an area with a higher frequency of earthquakes (like Southern California), in which case choosing to seismically retrofit your home makes good sense, even though broad nationwide statistics would indicate the risk of an earthquake is extremely low overall.

For many things, however, we take selective notice of low-risk events even if our microenvironment does not have an increased probability. When a plane crashes, we hear about it on the news, and it makes a big impression. The news gives it top billing, sometimes for days, with ongoing interviews of the families of the victims. The story can go on for weeks or months afterward with investigations, reports, and inquiries. Conversely, the news does not report a running total of all the flights each day that do not crash. Hollywood has made a number of movies about doomed flights, such as *Flight 93*, *The Horror at 37,000 Feet*, and *Terror in the Sky*, as well as many movies in which a plane crash figures prominently, such as *Cast Away* and *Final Destination*. Despite this perception, plane crashes are extremely rare; many more people die in car crashes every single day.

Car crashes seldom make the news (unless they were particularly horrific or involved a celebrity), and even then, they are covered only fleetingly compared with plane crashes. Car crashes do happen in movies, but we rarely see entire movies dedicated to a car crash. It is just a cause of a cool explosion or special effect that goes on in the background. Earthquakes may be more likely in Southern California than in other places, but plane crashes are not more likely when flying from Chicago to Florida than to other places. When my family thought about how we should get to Florida, images and memories of plane crashes were readily "available" in our minds, but car crashes were not, even though the risk of a car crash is much higher than that of a plane crash.

Because risk fits the form of a fraction, the way the availability heuristic affects risk assessment can be explained in terms of misperceiving the fraction. We pay attention to the top of the fraction (that which we happen to encounter, notice, or remember) and ignore the bottom of the fraction (everything else).

Assessing risk based on the association in one's mind is not necessarily a bad way of thinking if that is all the information we have. Giving full consideration to the data that are available (typically personal experience and stories) is certainly better than just randomly guessing. In modern times, however, humans often have access to sophisticated analyses of large quantities of accurate population-based data. Nevertheless, despite such information, humans tend not to seek these details. The availability heuristic becomes a problem when it is no longer the best approach, but we prefer it anyway, even over sets of data that would help us better assess risk, if only we paid attention.

Strikingly, it is not just an issue of failing to seek high-quality data—people even ignore high-quality data that is provided to them. When exposed to anecdotal evidence and statistical data that contradict each other, people tend to prefer the anecdotal evidence.[13] Public health messages around safe-sex practices to avoid sexually transmitted diseases are more effective when given as a testimony from a recognized person of the group being addressed than when presented as factual statistical evidence from robust epidemiological data.[14] The effectiveness of narrative information depends on the nature of the narrator and the specifics of the message; nevertheless, the phenomenon persists.[15] One might think that the less persuasive nature of statistical data is because the audience lacks particular expertise in the area being addressed. Even trained professionals, however, have shown a preference for anecdotal evidence over large data sets in their field of expertise, despite the data sets being high quality based on large sample sizes and with compelling statistical rigor.[16]

This is one explanation why so many people insist that the measles vaccine causes autism, when overwhelming evidence indicates that this is not the case.

The evidence suggesting that the vaccine causes autism encompasses stories, whereas the refuting evidence is supported by large carefully conducted scientific studies.[17] We evolved to find the former highly convincing; the latter just does not naturally resonate with us—and why would it? From an evolutionary point of view, we have gained access to robust population-based data only recently.

A professional risk assessor for an insurance company, someone whose job and focus are the accurate determination of the actual frequency at which things occur, may have an experiential basis (at least in the form of data they encounter), which is pretty close to the actual world. The rest of us get most of our information from our personal experience, the experience of the people with whom we speak or correspond (i.e., family, friends, and coworkers), the news media (in the particular forums that we seek out or encounter), Hollywood and entertainment, and in recent years, social media.

We extrapolate what we encounter on a personal level to an assumption of broader statistical frequencies. For example, people who watch television soap operas believe in a higher societal frequency of professions typically portrayed on soap operas (e.g., doctors and lawyers) and overestimate the frequency of other scenarios portrayed in soap operas (e.g., illegitimate children and divorce)[18] as well as in the increased prevalence of general affluence often associated with soap opera characters.[19] Similarly, people who see more advertisements for depression medications overestimate the prevalence of depression in society.[20]

The effects of the availability heuristic extend far beyond individual decision making—for example, this heuristic has profound effects on government decisions. The United States consists of approximately 350 million citizens, but legislative decisions are ultimately made by only 536 of these people (i.e., 435 representatives, 100 senators, 1 president). In this case, the personal experience of the legislatures and the chief executive may not be of much relevance to what makes good policy. Instead, what is relevant is what happens to the whole country, both in terms of general trends as well as in terms of different geographies and subpopulations around the country. For this reason, the government spends immense resources gathering and processing data and statistics from around the country and in a variety of categories.

In many cases, statistical data are used to excellent effect to promote the general welfare. For example, the implementation of seatbelt laws, the prohibition of texting while driving, and compelling warning labels on cigarettes. Some leaders, however, appear to make broad policy decisions, national and international, based on personal experience and what they have heard from others, or even worse, what they have read on a Twitter feed or heard commentators say on a particular network. They simply may ignore, or even be unaware of, the broader statistical data. In some cases, they may have distain for data collection and analysis. When such individuals affect policy, it amplifies the effects of the availability heuristic on a massive scale, afflicting many people.

One has to look no further than former President Trump as a prime example of immensely powerful people making broad decisions favoring anecdotal evidence over robust scientific data. Donald Trump often makes claims that appear to be in conflict with significant evidence to the contrary. Time and again, when asked to justify his belief, his response is that "there are a lot of people that think . . ." or "You know, a lot of people are saying . . ."[21] Some have suggested that this is a clever and calculated strategy to allow the spreading of conspiracy theories without directly supporting them, but rather by attributing it to things other people are claiming.[22] The case of Trump's belief in hydroxychloroquine and COVID-19, however, seems clear.

To be fair to President Trump, he had a reasonable basis to suspect, early on, that hydroxychloroquine had a chance to be an effective treatment based on the reported effects of chloroquine on the SARS virus, which is related to the virus that causes COVID-19.[23] On the basis of such background information, and as is appropriate, controlled studies were then performed, showing that hydroxychloroquine, in fact, had no effect on either preventing or treating COVID-19.[24] Yet, Trump remained hellbent on promoting the use of hydroxychloroquine— so much so that he claimed to be taking it. When asked what evidence he had that it worked, he said, "Here's my evidence: I get a lot of positive calls about it" and "Couple of weeks ago I started taking it because I think it's good. I've heard a lot of good stories."[25]

Of course, many legislators may understand all too well what the statistical data show, but they also make policies based on what appeals to the electorate, and the electorate forms opinions largely based on personal experience, news media, and social media feeds. Humans are storytelling animals who respond to the anecdotes and information received from speaking with other humans. Since President Ronald Regan's term, it has been common practice for presidents (of either party) to bring particular citizens to State of the Union speeches, have them stand up to be recognized, and in many cases, to justify policy arguments based on their stories. Using individual examples resonates with voters, whereas statistical arguments fall flat. We remember stories that we hear, but we are hard-pressed to remember facts, figures, and data analysis— the stories remain "available" to us in our minds and influence our thinking.

Circling back to my childhood trips to Florida. Had we wisely decreased the risk of death by choosing to drive rather than fly? One commonly hears that car travel is much more dangerous than air travel because the lifetime risk of dying in a motor vehicle crash in the United States is about 1/100 compared with the risk of dying in a plane accident, which is too low to accurately calculate.[26] Even this apparently mindful consideration of statistics and comparison of actual risk, however, makes an error of comparing two different fractions. The reason is that people fly much less frequently than they drive, and some people never fly at all, whereas many people have to drive, often for hours on a daily basis. Maybe our increased lifetime risk of dying in a car crash rather than in a plane crash is because we spend so much more time driving than flying? In addition, my family was making a decision regarding mode of travel for a specific trip of a defined distance. A better comparison is the risk of driving versus flying per miles traveled. Even in this case, the risk of dying in a car crash is 750 times higher than in a plane crash on a per-mile-traveled basis.[27] We had increased our likelihood of dying en route from Chicago to Florida by driving.[28]

I have seen the availability heuristic at play in my role as a physician. I have encountered patients who were morbidly obese late-middle-age males, who smoked four packs of cigarettes a day, paid little attention to their untreated diabetes, and rode a motorcycle without a helmet. But what they were really scared of, what worried them most, was that they might be killed by a terrorist. If their goal was to avoid bad outcomes, the availability heuristic was working solidly against them; they were missing all manner of opportunities to address the controllable risk of things likely to happen to them, but instead, they focused their energies on things that had an extremely low likelihood.

Obesity accounts for 5–15 percent of deaths each year in the United States, whereas smoking accounts for 18 percent.[29] The chance of being killed by a terrorist in the United States is 1 in 27 million (for domestic terrorists) and 1 in 3.7 million (for foreign-born terrorist), this latter number being higher following the attacks of September 11, 2001. The news occasionally may air a story on the thousands of people who die from diabetes or smoking each year, but typically it is a report by a medical correspondent in a low-key format on "a slow news day" or an article in a magazine, but it is not considered breaking news. In contrast, when terrorism does occur, we are bombarded with images and dialog for months or even years. To my knowledge, Hollywood has yet to release a thriller entitled *Diabetes*.

The availability heuristic is by no means restricted to noticing bad things; indeed, it likewise finds a place in predicting the frequency of good or desirable things. People who are exposed to news stories about lottery winners perceive the odds of winning to be much higher than they really are.[30] As such, they are more likely to spend money on the lottery, almost guaranteeing the loss of the money they spend. Las Vegas casinos spend so much money advertising the stories of winners, and strategically place winning slot machines near casino entrances, precisely so passersby will see other people winning and chose to come in the casino.

The availability heuristic is deeply seated in our minds. Even advanced education and extensive experience does not eliminate it. If a doctor recently had a patient with a certain disease, the doctor tends to overestimate the likelihood that other new patients also will have that disease.[31] Likewise, doctors undertreat severe pain with opioids, precisely when opioids should be used, because of the high publicity that opioid addiction gets. This is not to say, in any way at all, that opioid addiction is not a major problem or that opioids are not overprescribed in cases when they are not justified—they are a major health crisis and have led to much suffering and death. The fear of addiction, however, also leads to the underprescribing that results in much unnecessary suffering, because of the perceived likelihood of addiction.[32]

Summary

In this chapter, we explored how we act upon only a fraction of the information available in the world. Through limits of our sensory organs, we are capable of perceiving only a small fraction of the available information. Of the information that we can perceive, we notice only a small amount of it. Of what we do notice, we focus disproportionately on particular information and ignore much of the rest. Finally, of what we do focus on, we remember only a fraction of even that. This often can be a good thing. It allows a razor-sharp focus on the information that is important and allows us not to become overwhelmed with the deluge of information that otherwise might distract us from vital facts.

Our natural tendencies, however, become a problem when, through our focus, we miss additional information we should be aware of. Moreover, in modern times, when high-quality population-based data are available, data that if considered would help us make better decisions, we fail to seek it out. Even worse, we fail to recognize such data as meaningful and specifically ignore it, even when it is presented to us in easy-to-digest formats. This need not result from the purposeful manipulation by others, we do this on our own without being aware we have done so. That said, such tendencies also represent a pathway by which those who wish to manipulate us can easily do so, because we happily accept claims that distort the world in particular ways, because they resonate with the normal processes by which humans tend to think.

CHAPTER 3

CONFIRMATION BIAS

How Our Minds Evaluate Evidence Based on Preexisting Beliefs

C apital punishment is a polarizing political issue. Killing humans for the crimes they commit has a long and profound history. In the context of British law, one of the oldest operating legal systems, executions were at one time extremely common. By 1800, one could be executed for more than 200 different crimes, including something as trivial as wearing a disguise while trespassing or strong evidence of malice in a child (you read that correctly, not malice *towards* a child but malice *in* a child).[1] Since that peak, crimes for which one can be executed progressively decreased. Currently, no industrial nation executes its prisoners except for the United States, where it is the law of the land in 27 out of 50 states. Worldwide, 56 out of 195 countries have capital crimes and actually carry out executions.

The debate on capital punishment typically includes the question of whether or not it is a deterrent to crime. In other words, does capital punishment decrease the rate of the crimes to which it is applied? Consider your current view on this issue. The relevant data are complex.

With reference to capital punishment in the United States, a study by Kroner and Phillips compared murder rates for the year before and the year after adoption of capital punishment in 14 states. In 11 of the 14 states, murder rates were lower after adoption of the death penalty. This research supports a deterrent effect of the death penalty. In contrast, a separate study by Palmer and Crandall compared murder rates in 10 pairs of neighboring states with different capital punishment laws. In 8 of the 10 pairs, murder rates were higher in the state with capital punishment. This research opposes the deterrent effect of the death penalty. In light of these findings, what do you think now? How do these data affect your belief about whether or not capital punishment is a deterrent, and why? Take a moment and think about it.

This exercise is derived from a psychology experiment carried out at Stanford University in the late 1970s.[2] The study was performed on two groups of undergraduates who had been identified several weeks earlier by an in-class questionnaire regarding their preexisting beliefs. The first group supported the death penalty and felt it was a deterrent—the second group held opposite views. Subjects from both groups were mixed together and seated at a large table. The person running the experiment did not know which subjects belonged to which group. The subjects were each told that they would receive two index cards, chosen at random, from 20 studies on the deterrent effects of capital punishment. Each card would have the result from one study. Subjects were instructed to read the first study, assess if and how their view had changed, and then read the second study, again assessing if and how their view had changed (the subjects rated their beliefs on a numerical scale).

In reality, each of the subjects read descriptions of the same two studies, which were fictitious but were written to be "characteristic of research found in the current literature cited in judicial decisions."[3] The result of the experiment was that both groups increased their belief in their initial position after reading the cards. In other words, diametrically opposed views were both strengthened by the very same information, presented in exactly the same way. Importantly, this was not due to the inherent quality of the studies being described (i.e., one being more rigorous than the other), because the researchers found the same effect when they switched the outcomes of the fictional studies. It also was not due to the order in which the subjects read the studies; the researchers controlled for this as well.

How could the very same data simultaneously support opposite and mutually exclusive views? The subjects wrote down assessments of the studies they read, and their responses revealed a clear effect. Each group rated the research supporting their preconceived view as high quality and rated opposing research as low quality.[4] Moreover, it was not simply an issue of stating a preference. Subjects gave very specific reasons for why they favored some research over others, commenting on experimental design, time length of study, randomization of groups being compared, and number of independent variables. These are appropriate and legitimate scientific issues to be considered in research; however, it presents one problem. The subjects identified the virtues and flaws of the studies not as a function of the studies themselves, but as a function of whether or not the study's conclusions aligned with the subjects' preexisting beliefs.

We are describing a different effect than what was put forth in the first two chapters. In this case, the individuals were exposed to the identical data, but assessed it differently based on what they thought before they encountered it. This is a subconscious process that has been termed "confirmation bias," which has been described as "the seeking or interpreting of evidence in ways that are partial to existing beliefs, expectations, or a hypothesis in hand."[5] People are not objective observers of the evidence they encounter; rather, how we observe the world is influenced by what we already believe. At least to some extent, it's not that we believe what we see. Rather, we see what we believe.

If you think that your views are highly supported by the evidence that is available, and opposing views are not, then you might think again. This could be the case, but you likely would feel the same way regardless of whether or not this is true. Those who oppose your views likely have the same strength of conviction that their views are justified by existing evidence, while your views are not.

Although the term "confirmation bias" was not coined until the 1960s by Peter Cathcart Wason, confirmation bias has long been recognized as a human tendency. As early as the Peloponnesian War (431–404 BCE), historian Thucydides wrote: "For it is a habit of humanity to entrust to careless hope what they long for, and to use sovereign reason to thrust aside what they do not desire."[6] This tendency was still with us over 2,200 years later, as noted by Henry David Thoreau regarding seeking certain types of plants in the forest: "We cannot see anything until we are possessed with the idea of it and take it into our heads— and then we can hardly see anything else."[7]

Formal experimental study of confirmation bias did not begin until the 1950s. An outstanding and comprehensive review of this topic was written by Raymond S. Nickerson in 1998, and while progress in understanding confirmation bias has been made since then, one cannot do much better in capturing the depth and breadth of the issue.[8] A hallmark of confirmation bias is that evidence supporting a belief is given greater weight than that refuting a belief— one is not evenly weighing evidence. In Nickerson's words, "once one has taken a position on an issue, one's primary purpose becomes that of defending or justifying that position. This is to say that regardless of whether one's treatment of evidence was evenhanded before the stand was taken; it can become highly biased afterward."[9] Even more extreme is that people who encounter evidence contrary to their belief may not only discount the evidence but may even use the evidence to increase their belief in that which the evidence refutes.[10]

Anyone who is paying attention to the heated polemics of the political struggles in the United States cannot help but see the confirmation bias unfolding in real time. Hugo Mercier and Dan Sperber have specifically pointed out that people do not just seek out confirmation of any idea that happens to enter their heads. They are very good at seeking and finding disconfirming evidence for ideas contrary to their existing beliefs. For this reason, Mercier and Sperber prefer the term "myside bias," which seems appropriate to today's world.[11]

Watch an hour of news on the same night from sources that differ in their political dispositions (in the United States, these might be Fox News, CNN, and MSNBC). It's hard to believe they exist in the same world with identical events. This same phenomenon likely would be observed in any nation regarding different sources of information. In the words of Raymond S. Nickerson,

> Many have written about this bias, and it appears to be sufficiently strong and pervasive that one is led to wonder whether the bias, by itself, might account for a significant fraction of the disputes, altercations, and misunderstanding that occur among individuals, groups, and nations.[12]

One might have the more cynical view that some news outlets are purposefully biased and represent instruments of propaganda by puppet masters with specific agendas. Of course, this could be the case. Because of confirmation bias, however, this need not be the case to explain the differences in opinion. Of course, these options are not mutually exclusive; both are likely at play.

Confirmation Bias Is Unintentional and Agnostic to Self-Benefit

Analysis of human behavior and thinking has uncovered all manner of bias. Our common dialog contains much concern about bias toward race, religion, age, gender, ethnicity, and sexual preference (among a great many other things). Terms, such as prejudice and discrimination, are commonly used to refer to such biases. Confirmation bias, however, is fundamentally different in nature. Confirmation bias is not a belief. Rather, confirmation bias is a process by which we reinforce our beliefs—any beliefs—regardless of origin or accuracy.

Our initial beliefs come from a number of different sources (things we observe, things we read, things we are told, things we dream, things we reason, gut feelings and intuitions). As we live, we have ongoing experiences, and they may (or may not) line up with our beliefs. One might think humans adjust their beliefs based on ongoing experience, but with confirmation bias, we adjust our experience based on our beliefs. Thus, confirmation bias is central to the maintenance of essentially all beliefs, whatever their origins.

Confirmation bias is agnostic to the correctness or falsity of a belief. For those who hold erroneous beliefs, confirmation bias causes them to hold on to those beliefs despite contradictory evidence. For those who hold correct beliefs, confirmation bias makes them more confident in their views than evidence justifies. Of course, people who maintain their beliefs based on evidence are acting rationally—if data support an idea, then it is rational to believe that idea. This presupposes that the data are accurate and correct and that we consider and weigh the evidence appropriately. Confirmation bias basically ensures that even with accurate data, we do not weigh it appropriately, and our assessment of that data is unduly affected by preexisting beliefs.

All manner of people purposefully cherry-pick evidence that favors their preexisting point of view and then intentionally interpret the evidence in the most favorable terms. This *is not* confirmation bias. Rather, confirmation bias has a similar effect to cherry-picking data, but the person is entirely unaware that they are doing so, and all the while believe they are being balanced in their assessments of information. Cherry-picking is explored in detail in chapter 4.

Importantly, confirmation bias is not simply an issue of being self-serving, of favoring beliefs that benefit us and dismissing views that are to our detriment. Nor is it just an issue of defending cherished beliefs to which we have emotional attachments based on faith, tradition, or conviction. Such motivating factors certainly play a role in how humans evaluate belief constructs. In the words of Upton Sinclair, "It is difficult to get a man to understand something when his salary depends upon his not understanding it."[13] In contrast, confirmation bias attaches to essentially all beliefs, including those that are irrelevant or even harmful to the believer. Confirmation bias exists in the background of our cognition for evaluating essentially any evidence in the context of any belief, and it is present all the time.

Timing of Information and the Primacy Effect

Confirmation bias kicks in as soon as a belief is formed. Therefore, information that is encountered early on, which leads to a belief, has a much greater effect than information that is encountered later. When shown a sequence of 60 poker chips of different colors and asked to determine the frequency of different colored chips, people favored the trend that occurred in the first 30 chips even though the second 30 chips reversed the trend.[14] Whichever belief had the evidence to support it first was favored regardless of subsequent evidence. This has been termed the "primacy effect."

The primacy effect is durable, even in the face of contradictory evidence. In one study, participants were asked to identify an image in a picture. Initially, the picture was so out of focus as to make it unidentifiable, but subjects were asked to make a guess. Of course, most guessed incorrectly. They were then shown a series of the same picture slowly coming into greater focus. The final picture was focused enough that control subjects, who had never seen the early unfocused pictures, could easily identify the image. Those who had seen the early pictures, however, tended to continue to prefer their first guesses (formed from the unfocused picture) even when they later saw the focused pictures that showed an image different from their guesses.[15]

The old saying goes, "you never get a second chance at a first impression." This idiom is referring to the primacy effect. Once you make a first impression (good or bad), the cards are stacked to maintain it, regardless of subsequent evidence to the contrary.

Why Confirmation Bias Fits the Form of a Fraction

In many ways, like issues introduced in chapters 1 and 2, the fraction is an excellent analogy to consider certain properties of confirmation bias. Let us assume that a person has a belief and encounters 20 pieces of evidence relevant to that belief: 5 support the belief and 15 contradict it. Let's also assume that each piece of evidence is of equal quality. The percentage of information that supports the belief is 5/20 or 25 percent. All things being equal, it seems that a rational person should change their view, or at least weaken their convictions, because 75 percent of the evidence is inconsistent with the belief. Confirmation bias is such, however, that one may hold onto their belief despite a majority of evidence contradicting it, and this may even strengthen their belief. How would this happen?

As we learned with the death penalty example, this occurs when we exaggerate the quality of the supporting data and underestimate the quality of the refuting data. It also can be done in a qualitative fashion in which one just does not notice the evidence that goes against the belief—it simply never registers. In its extreme example, if one notices the 5 pieces of evidence that support the belief and fails to notice the 15 pieces that contradict it, the fraction of 5/20 (25 percent of evidence supports the belief) has been transformed into 5/5 (100 percent of evidence supports the belief).

One has thrown disconfirming evidence out of the fraction, similar to the no-true-Scotsman fallacy (described in chapter 1). All of the evidence supports the belief: because disconfirming evidence was excluded, it does not count as evidence. Who would not believe something that 100 percent of the evidence supports? Or one might take both approaches, simultaneously changing the quantity of the numerator or denominator and also changing how each is weighed with regards to quality. This dual, and very potent, approach is how confirmation bias can fully exert its effects.

Someone might hold the view that Muslim immigrants are terrorists, or at least more likely to be terrorists than anyone else. When the news reports an act of violence by a Muslim immigrant, then it is noticed—reports of violence by members of other demographics are just ignored. It goes much deeper than this, however. If an act of violence is perpetrated by a person with an Arabic-sounding name or with a brown or black skin complexion, it is counted as a data point of a Muslim committing an offense—regardless of the person's actual ethnicity, religion, or immigration status. Moreover, when an offense is committed by a person with this broad definition of being a Muslim immigrant, anything that causes disruption is considered terrorism. Suddenly, an American-born Hindu businessperson of Indian descent protesting at a political rally becomes a confirming case of how Muslim immigrants are terrorists, whereas non-Muslim Caucasians who *actually* blow things up (e.g., the Unabomber Ted Kaczynski, and Oklahoma City bombers Timothy McVeigh, and Terry Nichols) somehow are not counted as terrorists.

The problem is not limited to how people process the information that they just happen to come across. As we shall explore next, in the now-famous Wason 2-4-6 task, people tend to seek information and ask questions that serve to confirm their ideas and not seek information that may refute them. It is not just a quantitative and qualitative filter of the world one passively encounters, it is an active process that alters what information one is ever exposed to.

Two, Four, Six, Eight . . . Confirmation Bias Is Innate!

Peter Cathcart Wason was a British psychologist who first coined the term "confirmation bias" and described a famous and illustrative example called the "2-4-6" task.[16] A series of research subjects were provided with the numbers of 2, 4, 6 and were told that these numbers conformed to a particular rule. The rule was a relationship between any three numbers, of which 2, 4, 6 was just one example. The participants were supposed to figure out the rule. They could write down any three numbers they wanted and then would be told whether or not the numbers fit the rule. Subjects could do this as many times as they chose, using the feedback to refine what they thought the rule was. Once a subject thought they knew the rule, they could make a guess and would be told if they were right or wrong.

If they got the rule right, then the experiment ended. If they got it wrong, they could continue stating sets of three numbers (getting feedback as to whether or not they fit the rule) until they wanted to make another guess at the rule, and so on. In some ways, this is kind of like the game 20 questions. One person has a particular thing in mind, and the player can guess at its properties (getting "yes" or "no" feedback) to try to figure out what that thing is.

Most people initially wrote down three numbers that conformed to the rule they had in mind. For example, a common rule that came to mind was "increasing consecutive even numbers," and so a person would guess 12, 14, 16 to see if they got a positive "conforms to the rule" response. Presumably, their strategy was that if they got positive feedback from the examiner, then this would increase their confidence that they knew the rule. It was far less frequent for a participant to purposely guess numbers that did not conform to the rule they had in mind. After all, why would one do this? Answering this question is essential. Both the thought process and the logic construct differ between seeking confirmatory evidence and seeking rejecting evidence.

The 2-4-6 exercise is basically a model for exploring the world. It assumes that some rules actually exist, that we do not know what they are, and that we are seeking to identify them through experience. We guess at rules that are consistent with our experience and then we refine our guesses as we experience more things. This need not be a passive process; we can perform active experimentation—that is, tasks that are specifically designed to test the rules of the world we are living in.

Let's first examine the strategy of seeking confirmation. For many people, the first thing that comes to mind is "increasing consecutive even numbers"—after all, guessing 2, 4, 6 clearly conforms to this rule. The strong tendency is to then make a guess like 8, 10, 12. If the answer confirms that 8, 10, 12 "conforms" to the rule, then this increases confidence in the belief. Although this approach seems reasonable and follows common sense, it has some distinct problems. In particular, no matter how many experiments you run and get a positive result, you still cannot prove the rule is correct. But why not? This is the problem of evidence, confirmation, and induction most famously articulated by David Hume.

A classic textbook explanation is to consider someone who believes the natural rule that "all ravens are black." One might look at 100,000 ravens and find every one of them to be black. This is a lot of evidence to support the rule. But what if the very next raven turns out to be white?

Returning to our 2-4-6 exercise, one might believe the rule is "increasing consecutive even numbers" and then guess 4, 6, 8; then 10, 12, 14; then 20, 22, 24; and then 50, 52, 54 and so on. In every instance, the answer might be "conforms to the rule." In this case, one probably would become fairly confident that the rule is correct. But no matter how many instances of confirmation, the answer to the next guess of three increasing consecutive even numbers might be "no, it does not conform."

In contrast to the inability of positive instances, no matter how many, to absolutely prove a rule, a guess that gives a negative answer could indeed reject the rule, and it could do so with logical certainty.[17] A single white raven can reject the rule that "all ravens are black," and a single guess of three consecutive even numbers that "does not conform" could reject the "three-consecutive-even-numbers rule"—no matter how many previous examples conformed. As Albert Einstein is often quoted as having said, "No amount of experimentation can ever prove me right; a single experiment can prove me wrong."[18]

The importance of Wason's 2-4-6 study is that it appears to show the tendency of people to seek evidence that confirms their ideas rather than evidence that rejects them. For the above reasons, "confirmatory evidence" is less logically certain than "rejecting evidence."[19] Does this necessarily mean that seeking confirmatory evidence is a worse approach for figuring things out? Maybe. Of the subjects in Wason's study, those who tended to seek confirming examples with their three-digit guesses were less successful and took longer to figure out the rule than those who tended to seek rejecting examples.[20] In later studies, it was shown that when subjects were specifically instructed to guess at numbers that did not conform to the rule they had in mind, they then made faster progress.[21]

Wason made several other important and provocative observations. Of those whose first guess at the rule was wrong, more than half then stated their next three-number test as an instance of the rule that they just were told was incorrect. Three of the subjects who guessed incorrectly later made a second guess that invoked the very same rule as their first incorrect guess (albeit worded differently). Why humans have these tendencies is explored in more detail in chapter 11 (until then, simply consider that humans do have these tendencies).

The results of the 2-4-6 task have been reproduced extensively by numerous researchers, including other variations of the task. Importantly, some of these did not involve giving the initial example (e.g., 2, 4, 6). Instead, subjects just started guessing on their own and tended to fall into this very same pattern—that is, seeking confirmatory cases based on whatever their first guess happened to be.[22] The 2-4-6 task has been an amazingly fruitful experimental tool and has been used in multiple studies, in multiple contexts, and with many different particulars. Sixty years later (as explored next), no consensus has been reached on the precise interpretation of what the 2-4-6 task tells us about the underlying mechanisms of human cognition. What is clear and unequivocal, however, is that, at least under the conditions Wason defined, human cognition tends to function this way.

One, Five, Seven, Ten . . . Should We Interpret This Again?

The findings of Wason and others often are presented as strong evidence that humans are confirmation-seeking machines. That humans tend to behave as Wason described is clear, but did Wason interpret these findings correctly? In an insightful and thoughtful analysis of the issue, Professor Jonathan Evans went so far as to say, "There is no doubt that people do act in a manner which repeatedly confirms their hypotheses on the task and become convinced of their correctness."[23] As Evans goes on to explain, however, it is not clear that the tendency is motivated by a "confirmatory attitude." One cannot conclude that the human mind is "seeking to confirm" based solely on the behavior. If we cannot make this conclusion, then what other interpretations might there be?

If we believe the rule is "increasing consecutive even numbers," a guess of 8, 10, 12, appears to be an attempt at confirmation, whereas a guess at 1, 3, 7 appears to be an attempt to reject. This, however, is not necessarily the case: either guess can confirm and either guess can reject. The guess of 8, 10, 12 may be met with the answer "does not conform"; in which case, the subject should reject the rule in mind. A guess of 1, 3, 7 also may be met with an answer "does not conform." The latter guess at least provides some confirming evidence of the rule in mind, although it does not conform to the rule. Thus, guessing an instance that conforms to the rule in mind does not indicate whether or not the subject actually had a "confirmatory attitude." Here Evans makes the important distinction between "logical" and "psychological" confirmation.

Rules do not typically exist in isolation and an endless number of rules may fit the data we have. After all, although the rule we have in mind in our example certainly works for 2, 4, 6, so do a great many other rules. For example,

A. Increasing even consecutive numbers (our current belief)
B. Any three increasing numbers
C. Any three even numbers
D. The third number is the sum of the first two numbers
E. The second number is the average of the first and third numbers
F. Numbers that when spelled are four letters or fewer
G. And many other rules could apply. As long as one is willing to be creative, the sky is the limit. For example, "addresses at which Stephen Sondheim lived."[24]

Consider if the rule we have in mind is increasing even consecutive numbers. If we guess 4, 6, 8, as humans are prone to do, we find two possible outcomes. First, we may get an affirmative response: 4, 6, 8 fits the rule. This certainly confirms rule A (and also B, C, and E); however, this same result rejects D and F.[25] Alternatively, if we guess 4, 6, 8 and are told, no, it does not conform to the rule, then we can reject A, B, C, and E. This same answer now supports D and F. In contrast, if we guess 2, 3, 5, a positive result would render rules A, C, E, and F incorrect while confirming rules B and D. A negative result would reject B and D while supporting A, C, E, and F. Every guess has the capacity to confirm some rules and reject others.

In a subsequent study, subjects were told about two rules that were different (called DAX and MED) and that 2, 4, 6 conformed with DAX but not MED.[26] In this case, subjects were much better at figuring out DAX and MED than they were at the original 2-4-6 task. The subjects still behaved the same way—that is, they tended to seek positive instances. Because of two mutually exclusive hypotheses, however, every guess inevitably resulted in a rejection of either MED or DAX. Thus, deductive progress was being made through rejection as well as confirmation, regardless of what the psychological motivations actually may have been.

Importantly, not every attempt to confirm a hypothesis has the ability to reject other hypotheses under consideration. For example, having narrowed it down to just rules A and B, and then guessing 10, 12, 14 is a "nondiagnostic" guess, because it has no capacity to distinguish which rule is correct and which is wrong. The answer conforms to both rules. The answer still has the ability to reject both hypotheses if it is incorrect, but as per the cited studies, attempts at rejection do not appear to be the more common behavior. An example of a diagnostic guess is 4, 5, 6 because a positive result would reject A but not B.

The tendency toward nondiagnostic guesses also can be found even when two competing rules are mutually incompatible opposites. For example, a sobering and practical study was reported regarding people who preferred one product brand over another. When people were told an additional quality of the brand they favored, it increased their preference for the brand they liked, even when the quality was found equally in both brands.[27] Changing or reinforcing one's opinion based on nondiagnostic information is not logical, but it likely has widespread effects on each of us in our simple tasks of daily living.

Psychological Reinforcement of Confirmation

Humans have a psychological love of positive feedback, not just from other people, but from making progress on tasks of knowledge and understanding. I know of no better illustration of this than the following exercise with little kids. They are told they need to guess a secret number that is somewhere between 1 and 10,000. The question is asked "is the number higher than 5,000?" If the answer is "yes," then the kids cheer with enthusiasm. If the answer is "no," then the children give a groan of discouragement. Of course, the same information is gained either way; but our cognitive reflex is to favor the confirmation. Confirmation creates happiness in our brains. Is it any wonder that we may explore the world seeking confirmation? Who doesn't want little bursts of happiness?

Humans love to find answers to problems. Alison Gopnik, a professor of psychology at the University of California, Berkeley, likens the neurochemical feedback of puzzle solving to what we experience during sexual orgasm.[28] Indeed, when humans are placed in fMRI (functional magnetic resonance imaging) machines, which can scan the activity of different parts of the human brain in real time, it has been observed that our pleasure centers light up when we solve a reasoning task, that is, when we have an "Aha moment."[29]

It has been argued that the same brain centers are involved in "confirmation" for an idea and that "we actually get a dopamine rush when we find confirming data, similar to the one we get if we eat chocolate, have sex, or fall in love."[30] These same neurological pathways light up in behaviors such as gambling and drug abuse.[31] Notably, brain imaging scans on people who are given negative evidence against political parties and candidates they favor, and who then use confirmation bias to discount that evidence, clearly show activation of the brain in centers involved in emotional reasoning in contrast to other areas associated with reflective thoughtful reasoning.[32] We may be addicted to seeking confirmatory evidence because it feels good to find it. And if we can't find it, it feels just as good to use confirmation bias to misperceive the world guided by our preexisting beliefs.

Underlying human psychology reinforces preferences for confirmation in subtle but powerful ways. When given the choice between one-sided arguments versus those that explore both sides of an issue, people tend to consider the one-sided argument as the stronger argument and have more confidence in its conclusions.[33] As expertly explained by the research psychologist Professor Kevin Dutton, we favor "black-and-white thinking" and find discomfort in ambiguity or uncertainty.[34] People also tend to favor simple, positive, and confirmatory arguments and findings. Consider the one-sided sound bites in political ads and the relative lack of balanced or nuanced arguments. Politicians know their audience, and they use what works.

Humans even tend to use confirmation bias retroactively through a sad exercise in revisionist history. When selecting from a number of options, and having chosen what we think is the best option, humans subsequently denigrate what previously was the second-best choice to reassure ourselves about the choice we did make.[35] These are all "psychological confirmation," and they resonate with our intrinsic mental processes. As explored in this chapter, however, this is not "logical confirmation."[36]

Why Did Confirmation Bias Evolve in Humans?

The existence of confirmation bias seems to be a puzzling thing. What possible purpose could it serve? How could it ever be adaptive for our brains to blindly reinforce our existing beliefs, any belief, even self-destructive beliefs? We should consider that the approaches of Wason (and many others) describe how humans behave in psychology labs. This, however, is not where most people spend their time and certainly is not where humans evolved.

Rather, much of human thinking has evolved in the context of cooperative behavior and social contracts with other humans. Indeed, when Wason 2-4-6–like tasks are framed in a social context, then humans tend to do much better at the task (explored further in chapter 11). Moreover, emerging cognitive theories explain how confirmation bias (and heuristics in general) can have, at least at times, profound advantages over logical and reflective thinking (also explored further in chapter 11). Advantages are contextual, and although they may offer net benefits in some settings, that does not mean they cannot also be detrimental.

Summary

Confirmation bias is baked into human cognition and manifests in several different ways. The way we seek information makes it more likely that we encounter evidence that confirms our existing beliefs. Of the evidence we encounter, we tend to notice confirming evidence and ignore rejecting evidence. And of all the evidence we notice, we tend to assign a higher quality to confirming evidence and a lower quality to rejecting evidence. Confirmation bias attaches to whatever we believe first (the primacy effect), regardless of the origin or basis of the belief, and this bias then colors our observations from that point forward. Because confirmation bias generates new observations based on an initial belief, then these new observations can substitute for the basis of the belief even if the initial evidence that led to the belief is discredited. In this way, confirmation bias sets the bar quite high for what it takes to convince someone they are wrong. Confirmation bias is always running in the background of our cognition. In keeping with the theme of this book, confirmation bias can be understood using the form of a fraction. In evaluating an idea based on the percentage of evidence that supports it (supporting evidence/all evidence), our biased cognition alters the fraction by amplifying the numerator and diminishing the denominator.

CHAPTER 4

BIAS WITH A CHERRY ON TOP

Cherry-Picking the Data

C herry-picking is an insidious means of lying. It is not so blatant as simply stating something that is untrue. Rather, it is presenting a compelling argument for a falsehood by using data that are entirely accurate and correct, but just not using all of the data. Similar to the version of confirmation bias in which one notices only the evidence that supports a preexisting belief, cherry-picking selectively presents data that support a preexisting agenda. Unlike confirmation bias, which is subconscious, cherry-picking often is entirely intentional—and the perpetrator need not believe the result he or she is proclaiming.

Consider that you are in the marketing department of a large company and are attempting to understand consumer satisfaction of your product. You commission 10 different surveys of your product with different consumer groups. Nine of the surveys each show approximately 80 percent of people who purchased your product hated it and would not buy it again if their lives depended on it. One survey, however, showed a 55 percent approval rate. You are asked to give a presentation to the board of trustees for your company on consumer satisfaction with your product. You stand before them and say with a smiling face and a sincere tone that "in a recent survey we commissioned with a highly acclaimed firm, the majority of consumers approved of our product." Although you stated a true fact, the notion you communicated was false. You lied by omission—you selectively reported the one survey that was favorable and failed to mention the rest, giving the appearance that only one survey had been conducted. You cherry-picked the data.

Cherry-picking does not have to always focus on the minority of data to promote an erroneous view. One weekend in college, I went out for an evening with several of my friends. We had dinner, saw a movie, and then drank a bottle of vodka while watching the *X-Files* on television. The next day, while trying to ignore the waves of nausea I was experiencing by concentrating instead on the headache that felt like an alien would burst from my skull, my mom called my dorm just to say, "Hi honey, I know you are studying hard and I didn't want to bother you, but I wanted to make sure that you were doing laundry and had enough clean socks."

When she asked me what I had done the last night, I told her the truth: some friends and I had had dinner, seen a movie, and then come back to our dorm to watch television. Not only had I told her all true facts, I also had told her the majority of the facts—I left out only one small thing. Nevertheless, I had distorted the truth of the evening by omitting the regrettable vodka experience (I figured that what she did not know would not hurt her, even if it had hurt me).

It is precisely out of concern of cherry-picking information that the oath one takes, in many countries, when testifying in a court of law contains a phrase similar to "the truth, the whole truth, and nothing but the truth." If "the *whole* truth" weren't a part of that oath, then cherry-picking would be allowed.

Picking Cherries to Solve Climate Change Problems

Cherry-picking takes its most perverse form when politicians and pundits misrepresent scientific data—accurate and complete presentation of data is sacrosanct to scientific practice. Through cherry-picking, the populace can be misled to think that "scientific data" support the opposite result from what the data really show. When this occurs, opponents often call it out. Even well-articulated objections, however, seem to do little to stop the practice, and it is unclear to what extent people recognize this problem.

In his book *Not a Scientist: How Politicians Mistake, Misrepresent, and Utterly Mangle Science*, author Dave Levitan presents an excellent example.[1] Levitan focuses on the ongoing and venomous debate surrounding global warming. The issue at hand is the less controversial part of the debate. We are not considering whether the Earth is getting warmer because of human activity or whether the warming has any ill effects. Rather, we are simply asking whether or not the Earth is getting warmer at all.

Regrettably, this issue is so politically charged that you will almost certainly have a preexisting, and typically quite strong, opinion. Because of issues of confirmation bias explained in chapter 3, you therefore will view this issue through the filter of your existing beliefs (just as I do). For this reason, I ask that you try to step back and appreciate the example of how cherry-picking particular data misrepresented the larger body of evidence from which it was picked.

Climate scientists have been gathering data about the Earth's temperature for more than a century, and these data are compiled and tracked by NASA, among other groups. Like any dynamic system, the particular temperature of the Earth will vary from day to day, and from year to year, even for the exact same date or season. The temperature in Rochester, New York, on April 10, 2015, will naturally differ from April 10, 2016, and from April 10, 2017, regardless of whether the Earth is getting hotter, colder, or remaining the same temperature. It was on April 20, 2016, at a campaign rally, that Donald Trump noticed it was below average temperature on that day and famously quipped, "we need some global warming." One could argue this was just a joke, but the tactic is so widely used, it cannot be discounted as mere whimsy. This is obvious cherry-picking-type thinking. One particular cold snap is no evidence against global warming, just as a particularly hot week is no evidence for global warming. Rather, one has to look at averages over time, from year to year, to identify what is happening overall.

One way to correctly analyze the Earth's temperature is to compare the temperature on each date of a year with the average temperature of that particular date in recent years (typically the previous 30 years). The difference between a day and its historical average is called the "temperature anomaly." Careful attention to location and method is required because on any given day, the temperature may be different at different measurement stations (even of the same latitude)—for example, because of differences in elevation.

Consider the graph shown in figure 4.1, which provides data collected from land and ocean measurements since 1880.[2] In this case, each data point (black box) represents the temperature anomaly for that year; in other words, how much warmer or cooler the temperature is compared with a 30-year average. As predicted for any dynamic system, we find natural variation from year to year, which is why the line is zig-zagged (the curved line is a "smoothing" operation to assist in visualizing the trend over time).

This graph does not represent the temperature of the Earth; rather, it shows whether the Earth is warmer or cooler in a given year than average. So, from 1880 until 1940, the Earth was cooling. After 1910, the extent of cooling began to decrease, and in 1940, it first crossed the threshold from cooling to warming. The last time the Earth had a negative temperature anomaly was in 1976. In other words, the Earth has been warmer than a rolling 30-year historical average each and every year for the past 45 years.

Based on these data, in 2015, Senator Ted Cruz made the following statement:

The scientific evidence doesn't support global warming. For the last 18 years, the satellite data—we have satellites that monitor the atmosphere. The satel-

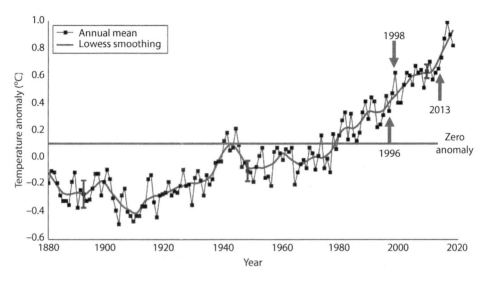

4.1 Global mean estimates based on land and ocean data.

Source: Adapted from J. Hansen, R. Ruedy, M. Sato, and K. Lo, "Global Surface Temperature Change," *Review of Geophysics* 48, no. 4 (2010). © John Wiley and Sons, used with permission.

lites that actually measure the temperature showed no significant warming whatsoever.[3]

In a separate interview with the *Texas Tribune*, referenced by Levitan,[4] Cruz made the following statement:

> The satellite data demonstrate that there has been no significant warming whatsoever for 17 years. Now that's a real problem for the global warming alarmists because all of the computer models on which this whole issue is based predicted significant warming, and yet the satellite data show it ain't happening.[5]

Cruz's statements have some truth to them (although very little), from a particular point of view. If we consider that the temperature anomaly in 1998 was plus 0.62°C and that in 2013 it was plus 0.65°C, then it is correct to say that there was no significant increase over a 15-year period (0.65 is not "significantly" larger than 0.62 from a statistical point of view). Although the data have been refined over time such that the exact range of years varies depending on which analysis is being used, the trend is the same. It is this time period to which Cruz is referring in his statement.

The problem with Cruz's analysis is that 1998 was a year in which the temperature anomaly was particular higher than the trend. Therefore, using that year as the baseline for comparison gives the appearance of no change. In contrast, the average trend over that same time is clearly still increasing.

By selectively focusing on only two points of data and ignoring data from all other years, Cruz provided a cherry-picked view that the Earth is not getting warmer. Had he widened his gaze by a single year (1997 is 0.47), or even narrowed his gaze by a single year (1999 is 0.4), then the same calculation would have shown a substantial increase (40 percent) over the same time period. Note that Cruz did not refute the data measurements; he accepted them. He could have said the data were incorrect—he did not. Rather, having accepted all the data as correct, he then cherry-picked data from two specific years and ignored the rest. In this case, his approach is not due to a cognitive error, but rather it has the particular intent of manipulating results to give the opposite answer of what is obvious when looking at the whole picture. In other words, he cherry-picked the data.[6]

Even if we were to accept Cruz's claim that the data did not increase over time, it is essential to remember what the numbers represent—not the temperature of the Earth, but how much warmer it is than on an average year (or the rate at which it is warming). By referring to these data and saying that "the satellites showed no significant warming whatsoever," Cruz actually was arguing that the rate at which the Earth is getting warmer is stable; however, the Earth is still getting warmer each year. This comment is akin to saying that because the rate at which your car is accelerating is constant your car is not speeding up. This approach indicates either a fundamental misunderstanding of what the numbers represent or a purposeful distortion of their meaning. Either way, when Cruz claimed that the numbers are stable, he basically stated that the Earth is indeed getting warmer each year, because the numbers reflect the amount of temperature increase and not the temperature. At best, Cruz was saying that the rate of warming is not increasing, but *not* that the Earth is not warming.

Again, you may not believe the Earth is getting warmer; however, should such be the case, your skepticism should not be based on the myopic and misleading analysis by Cruz. Even if the Earth is not getting warmer, even if NASA's data are fabricated and part of a conspiracy, this example is no less poignant. It is a clear case of distortion through cherry-picking.

Questioning if the numbers are correct and if data have been gathered accurately is part of good science. Accepting that the numbers are correct, but then purposefully distorting their meaning is anathema to science. It is this latter activity that Cruz enabled. It is a frequent instrument of manipulation that we should be aware of, guard against, and neither accept nor allow.[7] It is not my intention to pick on Cruz to the exclusion of others. I selected this example with Cruz because the attempted distortion is so painfully clear. Regrettably, cherry-picking is all too common and is perpetuated by multiple politicians and of all parties.

Cherry-Picking Seems Standard Practice in Politics

In the summer of 2012, the presidential campaign between then-incumbent President Barack Obama and challenger Mitt Romney was in full swing. As with any presidential election, a great many claims were made by the respective campaigns about the virtues of their candidate and the shortcomings of the opponent. This is good and proper as long as the claims are honest and legitimate—juxtaposition of candidates and debate of policies and performance should be part of our political discourse. As is sadly typical, however, both sides distorted information to favor their own candidate. Notably, both Barack Obama and Mitt Romney received equivalent "Pinocchio Scores" from the *Washington Post* "Fact Checker" column.[8]

Employment was a major issue in the 2012 campaign. Consider figure 4.2, which shows the size of the labor force (i.e., the number of full-time employed people, in thousands), by month, from 2007 to 2012 according to the U.S. Department of Labor and Statistics.[9] Looking at the graph, it is easy to find the Great Recession of 2008 when job loss was a major driving force. On January 1, 2008, more than 121 million jobs were reported. Two years later in January

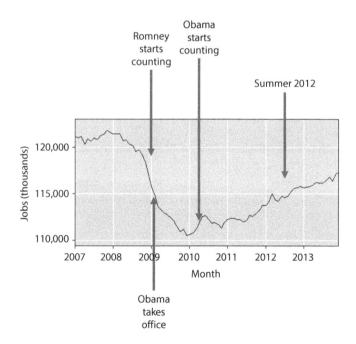

4.2 Size of the U.S. labor force from 2007 to 2012.

Source: Adapted from data by the U.S. Department of Labor and Statistics.

2010, fewer than 111 million jobs were reported and 10 million jobs had been lost in just two short years.

When assessing his own record on jobs, Obama claimed: "Over 4 million jobs [had been] created in the last two years." In contrast, referring to Obama's record, Romney claimed: "He has not created jobs." Who was right in these seemingly incompatible claims? Technically, they both were.

Romney started counting in January 2009, which basically was when Obama took office. By this measure, which captures all of President Obama's first term, Romney's claim is correct: there were fewer jobs in the summer of 2012 than when Obama took office. In contrast, Obama started counting in March 2010, more than one year into his presidency and after job numbers had bottomed out. There were four million more jobs in the summer of 2012 than in March 2010.

Unlike the egregious distortion of information that Cruz engaged in with global temperature anomalies, at least with Obama and Romney, one could make a philosophical argument. Why did Obama start counting in March 2010? Well, one could argue that whatever policies President Obama put in place could not be expected to start working right away: the economy was losing jobs so rapidly when Obama took office that it was unfair to start counting then. Alternatively, it seems fair for Romney to say that if we are going to count the effect Obama's presidency had on jobs, you count from his inauguration forward: it was all on his watch.[10] More likely, the real reason that each campaign selected the starting point they did is because the outcome favored their candidate.

Summary

In this chapter, we identified a specific type of distorting information that fits the form of misrepresenting the fraction. For any body of information, the percentage of information supporting a view can be represented by the fraction (supporting evidence/all evidence). By selectively presenting only the supporting evidence, and ignoring the rest of the evidence, one is distorting the fraction—that is, one is cherry-picking information.

Cherry-picking can be accomplished by different approaches. It can take the form of showing some data points and ignoring others, such as reporting only one out of a number of different surveys. It also can take the form of showing only specific time frames, as in the example of job creation. Cherry-picking can take the form of specifically selecting two specific time points out of a broader trend line, in which the difference between the time points does not represent the actual trends, as Cruz did with global warming. Cherry-picking does not have to result in a conclusion that is the opposite of what is really the case, it also can be used to exaggerate the extent to which something occurred—that is, the thing really did happen just not to the degree the cherry-picked data indicate.

As long as one is selectively presenting some data and omitting other data, with no legitimate reason for doing so, and with the intent of distorting reality, then one is guilty of cherry-picking.

PART II

THE FRACTION PROBLEM IN DIFFERENT ARENAS

CHAPTER 5

THE CRIMINAL JUSTICE SYSTEM

As of the time of writing this book, U.S. society is in the throes of an upheaval around a seemingly endless string of the killing of unarmed civilians by police officers. From 2015 to 2020, approximately 1,000 Americans were killed by police officers each year. In a particular period, reported by the *Washington Post*, police killed 2,532 Caucasians, 1,322 African Americans, and 925 people of Hispanic descent—clearly more Caucasians were killed than anyone else.[1] It seems like the police are biased against white people. After all, more white people are killed each year than other groups. But this is just the top of the fraction—and it is easy to see how focusing only on the numerator leads to the type of error described in part 1.

To compare between groups, one needs to consider the rate, not the absolute number. The rate of killing is 32 African Americans per million, 24 Hispanic Americans per million, and 13 Caucasian Americans per million. Overall, these minorities are killed at more than four times the rate of Caucasians.[2]

In recent years, given the proliferation of digital recording by bystanders, we now face the irrefutable evidence of what has long been the sad reality of the United States—a reality that has been well known by minorities for a long time. Some police officers act in a way that amounts to summarily executing citizens—and the citizens who are murdered in this fashion are disproportionately minorities.

Of course, one has to be careful not to fall prey to the availability heuristic detailed in chapter 2. More Caucasians than minorities are killed by police each year, but the killing of minorities generally receives far more news coverage.

Thus, people likely overestimate the extent by which minorities are killed at a greater rate by police. However, just because heuristics sometimes get things wrong, does not mean they don't also get things right. The availability heuristic may cause us to have an exaggerated view of excess killing of minorities, but careful analysis of the data confirms that minorities are killed at 4 times the rate as Caucasians.[3]

The fact that minorities are killed by police at a greater rate does not, in and of itself, prove that there is institutional or even individual racism. There may be other confounders that explain what is happening. For example, perhaps police kill people they encounter at an equal rate regardless of race, but police just have much more contact with minorities. According to the U.S. Department of Justice, this is not the case. Police are equally likely to initiate contact with African Americans vs. Caucasians (11 percent of each). However, once police do initiate contact, police either threaten or actually use physical force over twice as often with African Americans (5.2 percent) as with Caucasians (2.4 percent).[4] Does this demonstrate racism? Perhaps, but not necessarily. Another possible confounder is age. The average age of African Americans is 27; the average age of Caucasians is 58.[5] Perhaps minorities are killed by police more frequently simply because young males are most commonly killed, and minorities happen to currently have a higher frequency of young males. However, this alone cannot account for the extent of increased killing of minorities. What one really has to ask is, all other things being equal, do the police treat minorities differently, and if so, why?

The above data do not mean that most police officers are not good and honorable people who risk their lives every day for the safety and well-being of others. Of the more than 680,000 police officers in the United States, only a small number are involved in killings of civilians, and even fewer in unjustified killings. That most police officers are good and honorable people, however, does not erase the horrific acts done by those who are not, nor does it speak to underlying issues of institutional racism. To understand how unequal treatment of minorities is woven into the system, one must dig deeper.

Hiding of Bias Through Categorization

The Federal Bureau of Investigation (FBI), which is responsible for monitoring and preventing domestic terrorism in the United States, categorizes terrorists into different groups. Before 2017, white supremacists and far-right militant groups were two separate and distinct categories. Although white supremacists and far-right militant groups were responsible for the majority of terrorist acts, the FBI was focusing its resources on investigating other groups linked to racial and societal minorities.[6] When considering why resources were not focused on the groups most responsible for terrorism, it has been suggested that this is just another manifestation of institutional racism that is baked into our system. The increased scrutiny of groups based on racial affiliation is independent of the risk they actually represent.

In an attempt to draw attention to this issue, Senator Dick Durban introduced a bill called the Domestic Terrorists Act in 2017. This law requires the FBI to report how resources are devoted to monitoring different groups according to how many people the groups kill. According to Michael German, a former FBI agent and whistleblower, the FBI responded to the Domestic Terrorist Act by combining the categories of white supremacists and "black identity extremists" into a single group. German claims that the FBI did this specifically to hide the fact that they were spending far less on investigating white supremacists and far-right militant groups than they should.[7]

This is an example of changing the appearance of an action by altering a fraction. It is the opposite of the no true Scotsman fallacy described in part 1, wherein one artificially increases a percentage by kicking datapoints out of the fraction. In this case, one is adding datapoints to dilute and obfuscate important information. One can no longer distinguish resources spent on investigating different groups of people as they are blended together. The process of recategorization makes it impossible for a person to determine resources spent on particular categories.

Of course, we cannot really know the FBI's intention in making this recategorization. It may very well have been for a separate and less sinister reason than suggested by Michael German, but perhaps not. Whatever the intent may be, this case serves as a potent example of how changing the categories that a fraction contains can make the world look quite different than it really is. Regrettably, this is just the tip of the iceberg. Similar considerations can be used to evaluate computer algorithms that, by removing humans from the equation, have been heralded as a specific remedy to human bias. But are they?

Big Data and Big Data Policing: How Computer Algorithms Can Both Hide and Amplify Bias

One of the buzzwords of recent years has been the concept of "big data." Big data is defined as expansive and massive data sets, gathered from multiple sources, that computers can analyze to identify correlations and connections that humans could not identify on their own. Big data approaches can be used for multiple purposes, but the form we most likely are familiar with is the advanced systems of product advertising.

Many of us receive advertisements for different products on our Amazon, Facebook, or Google accounts that clearly are tailored to us. Sometimes it is obviously a result of our own actions: you purchase something online and ads for similar items pop up, often immediately. Big data also uses information we never intentionally provided. Some of this information is about others to whom we are connected in some way.

Advertisements are pushed our way because of what people with our particular characteristics tend to purchase. These factors work together to allow big data algorithms to predict how we likely will spend money. For example, you may be Facebook friends with a person, who is Facebook friends with another person, who is part of a social cluster that, based on their characteristics, is more likely to be interested in energy-efficient humidifiers that look like Pokémon characters. As such, you get advertisements for a Squirtle humidifier that runs on potato batteries.

Of course, even the all-powerful supercomputer in the cloud can get things wrong. In the early days of Netflix, my child (five years old at the time) and I shared an account. The algorithm to find movies "suggested for me" treated us as a single person, and it appeared to be searching (albeit unsuccessfully) for a bizarre film that was a historical documentary of the American Civil War but that was cast entirely with the residents of Ponyville and Canterlot, preferably staring Twilight Sparkle, Rainbow Dash, and Princess Mia Mora Cadenza.

Big data often has been billed as a process by which human bias can be decreased, if not eliminated. Afterall, a calculating computer devoid of a human mind also should be devoid of human prejudice. The sad reality is that our data are deeply contaminated with bias from multiple sources (human and otherwise). Therefore, the output of our big data algorithms is likewise contaminated. As Tom Lehrer once quipped, "Life is like a sewer. What you get out of it depends upon what you put into it."[8]

Perhaps more important, the way algorithms are used can ensure that future data also will be collected in a biased fashion. In other words, big data approaches can perpetuate, and even amplify rather than decrease bias, and can do so in a way that is hidden and unknown even to those using the big data–based systems. How exactly does this occur?

A major area in which big data is both of particular interest and considerable concern is its use by police departments to target crime. Author Guthrie Ferguson explores this expertly in *The Rise of Big Data Policing: Surveillance, Race and the Future of Law Enforcement*.[9] Law enforcement is combining crime statistics from multiple sources and using big data computer algorithms to predict things such as (1) where certain types of crimes are more likely to occur; (2) the characteristics of people who are more likely to commit a certain crime; (3) at what time (month, day, and time of day) crimes are most likely to occur; (4) what the characteristics of victims are likely to be; and (5) what types of items are most likely to be stolen or vandalized (e.g., the adjusted risk of a car being stolen based upon color, make, and model).

In concept, the approach being used is nothing new. Police departments always have known some neighborhoods have higher rates of crime, some individuals are more likely to commit crimes, and some circumstances require more police attention than others. Certain behavioral traits correlate with criminal behaviors, and therefore, it is reasonable for police to pay more attention to people acting in certain ways. When predicting where something may be in the future, it is reasonable to search for it where it has been in the past (all other things being equal). The inevitable downside is that this approach results in different treatment not of people who actually are criminals, but rather of all people who have traits that correlate with criminal behavior, even if they are entirely honest and law-abiding individuals. Big data massively amplifies this effect, giving police a new metric by which to focus on certain people with certain traits.

Let's consider the issue of predicting who is most likely to commit a crime. The precise details of many big data algorithms are kept secret, but they are known to contain some obvious characteristics, such as previous arrests or convictions, being on parole, and known association with others who have been convicted of a crime. But what does "known associations" mean? Is being a neighbor or living on the same block enough? How about attending the same school? How about just being related? For example, in a database of gang members that has been used in California (called CalGang) the criteria for a person to be entered into the database include the following:

1. Subject has admitted to being a gang member.
2. Subject has been seen associating with documented gang members.
3. Subject is known to have gang tattoos.
4. Subject has been seen frequenting gang areas.
5. Subject has been seen wearing gang dress.
6. In-custody classification interview.
7. Subject has been arrested for offenses consistent with usual gang activity.
8. Subject has been seen displaying gang symbols and/or hand signs.
9. Subject has been identified as a gang member by a reliable informant/source.
10. Subject has been identified as a gang member by an untested informant.

To be entered into the database, a person must fulfill two of these criteria. On the surface, this may seem quite reasonable. Consider, however, that a person simply may live in a neighborhood in which gangs are common or present and also may talk to people he or she lives near and likely runs into. This alone would be sufficient to fulfill the second and fourth criteria. Does this mean that anyone who lives in a part of town that has gangs and has reasonable social contact with people living near them may be classified as being in a gang? If a gang moves into your neighborhood, and you cannot afford to move (or simply choose not to), you are guaranteed the designation of frequenting a gang area. What if the term "seen associating with" means simply living in the same building with, standing near each other on a street corner waiting for the crossing light, or having been seen near each other in a park on a summer day? As an example of the absurdity of possible errors, the above referenced CalGang database listed 42 infants as gang members because they fit two criteria.[10]

The real problem, however, is how these databases are used. Los Angeles police have purposefully entered false information about certain individuals, resulting in the Los Angeles Police Department being officially blocked from entering data.[11] But this is not the major problem that we are considering here: the use of databases like CalGang is problematic even if used exactly as designed, by entirely honest actors, and with 100 percent accurate data.

Police need "probable cause" to arrest someone or search for evidence, which is knowledge of certain "facts" that would lead a reasonable person to believe a crime is being committed or illegal contraband will be found. In contrast, to briefly detain, question, or even frisk someone, police need only to have "reasonable suspicion," which is based on a police officer's experience as to what personal traits and circumstances make suspicion sufficiently justifiable. This is a vague definition, which basically means that if something looks suspicious, based on an officer's experience, that is enough for the officer to act.

Each officer will have different experience, with different accuracies and biases, and all of these experiences are part of the legal criteria by which someone can be stopped and frisked by police. As a counterbalance, criminal defendants can always challenge a police officer's claim to having "reasonable suspicion." But what would it mean if being on a big data list was sufficient cause for a police officer to frisk someone regardless of what they are doing, even if nothing else justifies reasonable suspicion? What would it mean if merely being on the list resulted in increased surveillance and scrutiny? What would it mean if being on the list meant that one was prosecuted more often and more aggressively, and maximum penalties always were sought? Now, remember that someone may be on the list just because of where they live. So, solely because of your address, you can be frisked, be put under surveillance, and be more likely to be prosecuted while facing larger penalties. Frighteningly, in some cases, this is precisely how big data policing is being carried out.

Big data algorithms can be used to generate a "heat list" of specific individuals more likely to be either perpetrators or victims of crime. Such lists can have impressive accuracy; for example, in one time period, about 80 percent of shooting victims in Chicago were on the city's heat list before the crimes actually occurred.[12] A number of strategies to use heat lists exist, including (1) getting people on the heat list to attend (or phone into) community events that inform them they are on the list and what it means; (2) sending "custom notification letters" accompanied by a personal visit from law enforcement and social services; and (3) a broader approach that also includes increased provision of social service, counseling, and health care (to address health issues including mental health).[13] This approach can be combined with increasing public safety personnel and investment in physical infrastructure (e.g., fixing streetlights) in high-risk locations where people included on the heat list are located. Some departments have advocated the "bad apple approach": when people from the heat list are arrested, they are prosecuted as vigorously as possible with the highest possible penalties (even for petty offenses). The idea is to remove "bad apples" from society to the degree possible.

The extent to which these interventions actually work to decrease crime, and what their side effects may be, remains a matter of study and debate. Perhaps not surprisingly, a combination of these approaches appears to work best. The important issue for our discussion, however, is how use of big data heat lists affects the types of errors we defined in part 1 on this book.

Building on an example Ferguson provides, consider two young teenagers: one lives in an underprivileged inner-city environment, and the other lives in an affluent and socioeconomically privileged community.[14] Both have just turned 18 years old; the former is entering the workforce, and the latter has just enrolled in a private university. Both want to make some additional money; the former wants to make ends meet, and the latter wants to earn extra spending cash. Both tried cocaine during high school and know someone they can purchase it from. Both decide to buy cocaine, cut it, and sell it for a profit.

The underprivileged teen may wind up on a "heat list," simply because of where he or she lives, and this teen is more likely to be stopped and frisked at random regardless of actions. The affluent teen is practically immune from such capricious searching. Even though neither teen has any criminal record, and even if both teens are engaged in the same behavior, the underprivileged teen is more likely to be searched (and thus caught) than is the privileged teen.

Moving past the issue of differential scrutiny, consider what happens if both teens are caught by police. The underprivileged teenager would be arrested, lose his or her job, and enter the criminal justice system. In many cases, the teen either pleads guilty or is convicted—either way becoming a felon. If the teen is incarcerated, his or her list of associates who have criminal records now explodes. After prison (or instead of incarceration), the teen then enters the parole system and is further entered into big data systems. This lowers the threshold for being stopped and frisked by police even further, without doing anything illegal or even suspicious—just being on the heat list is enough.

In stark contrast, the affluent university student is more likely to be caught by campus security, recommended for some form of disciplinary action, undergo counseling, and reenter the mainstream student path without any public record of the transgression. Basically, the affluent teen faces few to no consequences. Even if the affluent student were caught by police and arrested, the likelihood of being prosecuted is lower as a result of not being on the heat list. This teen is not on the list simply because of where he or she lives. Even if prosecuted and convicted, the sentence may be lighter because of not being on a heat list.[15] Thus, with each teen having performed the same act (and no other acts), the outcomes are likely to be completely different based upon differential treatment by law enforcement.

With regard to the plight of the underprivileged teen, one might argue that had the teen not broken the law then nothing would have happened to him or her. This may be true, but it is irrelevant to the question of unequal treatment. Rather, for this discussion, we must focus on the fact that both teens had identical actions. For the underprivileged teen, the Fourth Amendment guarantee to not be subjected to unreasonable search and seizure meant less to begin with, and was then highly eroded going forward, a problem greatly amplified by big data approaches. For the affluent teen, the opposite occurred. The teens were identical in action, but were treated differently under the law.

How does this fit into the type of errors defined in part 1? The system specifically seeks out incriminating evidence more frequently on the underprivileged teen than on the affluent teen. This is analogous to confirmation bias because one is seeking information to confirm a person's criminality differently and also interpreting it differently, based upon a pre-existing belief. This bias is built into big data policing (as a joint result of the nature of the algorithm, and the policy of acting on it). A person's actual criminality is a fraction in which their criminal actions constitute the numerator and everything they do is the denominator.

In this example, both teens were identical in their behavior—they both had the same criminality fraction. More information was generated on the underprivileged teen (frequent searching and frisking), which led to a higher likelihood of a hit. Then, based upon this hit, the confirmation bias was amplified further, by moving the teen up the heat list, resulting in even more scrutiny and searching.

If two people had a criminality fraction of 1/100 (e.g., possessed cocaine one out of every 100 days), and the first person was searched 25 out of every 100 days, but the second was searched only once every 100 days, who would be more likely to be busted? It is that simple. Big data policing and heat lists make this a reality. For criminal prosecution, only the "hits" matter (i.e., numerator). If someone is searched and found to have cocaine, it really does not matter how frequently they were searched and did not have cocaine. The defense of "yeah, I deal cocaine, but not very often" would not likely be effective.

Although this is a theoretical example for illustrative purposes, its real-life manifestations are painfully clear. It has been well documented, under multiple circumstances, that even in cases in which Caucasians possess contraband at a greater frequency than do minority individuals, minorities are searched and arrested at substantially higher rates.[16] This occurs because law enforcement focuses more on minority populations, who are stopped and frisked more often, and are prosecuted more aggressively. This has always happened, long before heat lists, but big data policing and heat lists only exacerbate it further.

Note that we have changed our focus from "underprivileged" to "minority." Regrettably, on average, minorities constitute a greater percentage of underprivileged individuals than their percentage in the overall population. This is a significant fact. Although minority status may be legally excluded as an allowable criteria for heat lists, living in an economically depressed area is an allowable criteria. By focusing on economically depressed areas that contain a disproportionally high percentage of minorities, one is essentially using big data to make being a minority a criteria for inclusion on a heat list, by association. Minority status may always have been considered by some police in assessing what constitutes reasonable suspicion, and this has never been just. Big data policing algorithms almost certainly do this, and as such, they amplify or create bias (or both). This practice results in depriving minorities of their Fourth Amendment rights. It is different treatment under the law and it is but one example of how racism is institutionalized and baked into the system.

This discussion is meant to highlight the observational errors baked into big data analysis. It is not a comment on whether big data policing works to reduce crime, and even if it does, how to manage the abuses and biases to which it leads. In all fairness, to calculate the full benefits and potential detriments of big data policing, one must consider that big data also is used to monitor the police. Big data algorithms can predict variables (person, place, situation, time) when police are more likely to abuse civilians. Thus, in some cases, big data policing is policing the police.[17] Of course, there will be biases in this approach as well, based on how data on police are gathered, processed, and acted on.

Big data, at least in the way it is currently being used, is no remedy to human bias. Because of how these systems are designed and implemented, big data can exacerbate the existing human bias. This bias occurs in the absence of a human cognition. Even a silicon-based computer processor can have a confirmation bias, if it is programmed and used in a particular way, as currently happens to be the case.

Juries Convicting the Innocent

One of the most crucial fact-finding bodies in the world is the jury serving on a criminal trial. This group of people (typically 12) is charged with weighing the evidence in a case fairly and returning a verdict of guilty or not guilty. The jury's decision determines whether the accused is fined, deprived of their liberty, or even deprived of their life. What could be a more important evaluation of evidence than that? One particular manifestation of misunderstanding frequency and probability in jury trials has been appropriately named "the prosecutor's fallacy," and it has been a source of misjustice in the U.S. jury system.

Perhaps the most famous real-life example of the prosecutor's fallacy is a well-known case *People v. Collins*.[18] The victim in this case was a woman named Juanita Brooks, who was assaulted in Los Angeles by a person she described as a "blond-haired woman dressed in dark clothing." A separate eyewitness saw the assailant running away, corroborated that she had blond hair, and added that she had a ponytail and that a black male with a beard and mustache picked her up in a yellow car and drove off. Janet and Malcolm Collins were subsequently arrested by police because they matched the combined characteristics described by the victim and the witness.

Unfortunately for the prosecution, neither the victim nor the witness could pick either of the accused out of a lineup. Thus, the main thrust of the prosecution's case was that the accused had all of the characteristics identified by the victim and witness, and after all, what were the odds of that? It is probably fairly rare for mathematicians to get to be star witnesses, but this case was the exception. A mathematician explained to the jury that the odds of any two independent things occurring together was the probability of one event multiplied by the probability of the other. For example, the odds of a first coin flip being heads is 1/2 and the odds of a second flip being heads is 1/2, so the odds of two flips in a row being heads is $1/2 \times 1/2 = 1/4$ (or a 25 percent chance). If you flip a coin twice, you will only get two heads one in four times you flip both coins.[19]

Using this principle, testimony was given that the odds of someone in Los Angeles at that time owning a yellow car was (1/10), being a male with a mustache was (1/4), being a female with a ponytail was (1/10), being a female with blond hair was (1/3), being an African American male with a beard was (1/10) and being an interracial couple was (1/1,000). By multiplying each of these probabilities together, the odds of one couple having all six traits was estimated to be 1/12,000,000. Testimony was given that, therefore, there was only a 1 in 12 million chance of the accused not being the individuals who committed the crime. The jury convicted based upon these probabilities exceeding reasonable doubt.[20]

You may (or may not) feel that only a 1 in 12 million chance of being innocent is beyond all reasonable doubt, but that is not the question. Rather, the question is whether this type of reasoning is correct with regards to the probability argument? Let us stipulate that all of the probabilities of individual events were correctly estimated, that the variables were indeed independent, and that the eyewitness observations were correct.[21] If this is the case, then the mathematical argument certainly sounds reasonable. Regardless of how it sounds, however, it is fundamentally incorrect.

For couples who do have these traits, the odds of observing each of the stated traits in any random couple is not the same as the odds that they are the guilty party. Let's say that you were in a bar and a 20-something guy named Tim DeNouski threatened your life and then walked away. After you filed a complaint with the police, they did a search of all the names in New York and identified eight Tim DeNouski's between the ages of 20 and 30. So, the police went to the first name on the list and took him into custody. When they put him in a lineup, you couldn't pick him out, but never mind that, the police charged him anyway. Afterall, his name was Tim DeNouski.[22]

In the trial, they argued that since only 1/1,000,000 people in New York is named Tim DeNouski then the odds that he is not the guilty party are only 1/1,000,000. Or, in terms of the Collins case, because only 1/12,000,000 couples have the traits described by the witness, then the chance that the accused couple did not commit the crime is only 1/12,000,000. In actuality, 1/1,000,000 is the odds of arresting a random New Yorker and having it be someone named Tim DeNouski. Because the police first narrowed their search to people known to be named Tim DeNouski and arrested one of them at random, and because eight Tim DeNouski's live in New York, then the odds of the arrested man being guilty is only one in eight (1/8). In other words, his odds of being innocent is seven in eight (7/8)—a far cry from only 1/1,000,000. The prosecutor's fallacy is thinking the odds of the arrested man being guilty are 1/1,000,000 when they are really 1/8.

Ultimately, on appeal, the California Supreme Court overturned the conviction on the Collins case because of a number of different problems with the mathematics, one of which was that the court recognized the prosecutor's fallacy.[23] In his book *Innumeracy*, John Allen Paulos analyzes the Collins case and calculates the actual probability of Collins having been guilty to be a one in eight chance (in other words, a seven in eight, or 87.5 percent chance of being innocent)—just like Tim DeNouski. This is because, just like Tim DeNouski, only eight people had all the traits used to identify the accused party in the Collins case. So, having arrested one of them (with no other evidence), there is a one in eight (1/8) chance that they are guilty—or a seven in eight (7/8) chance that they are innocent. This new probability seems to fall far short of "beyond all reasonable doubt."

For false convictions to occur because of the prosecutor's fallacy, no prosecutorial misconduct is required. Both the prosecutor and the jury may "innocently" make this error as a common human cognitive mistake, which occurs because of our erroneous intuitions about probability. If the defense is either unaware of the fallacy, or is unable to explain it to the jury in convincing terms, then this problem can (and has) occurred. Thankfully, at least in the Collins case, the appeals court recognized the problem and reversed the conviction, although this did not prevent the original error from having been made. Rather, this special case of misunderstanding probability (by a professional mathematician no less), resulted in innocent citizens being deprived of their freedom by the state without sufficient evidence—both victimizing the wrongly convicted and allowing the actual guilty parties to remain free.

Summary

In keeping with the theme of this book, particular forms of bias in our criminal justice system have been explored—focusing on some that fit the form of rates, probability, or frequency. As detailed in part 1, these can be understood in the form of a fraction, which helps us appreciate how manipulation of the fraction (as in big data policing) or how mistaking one fraction for another (as in the prosecutor's fallacy), can have severe effects. This in no way encompasses all bias, individual or institutional, at play with regards to criminal justice. Other causes and manifestations of bias inherent in the U.S. criminal justice system are outside the scope of this work.

CHAPTER 6

THE MARCH TO WAR

On March 19, 2003, the United States of America and the United Kingdom (along with certain allies) invaded Iraq in what Americans refer to as the Iraq War or the Second Gulf War. Then–president of the United States George W. Bush led the charge. The current discussion is not an analysis of whether or not Saddam Hussein was an evil man; clearly, he was. This also is not an analysis of whether or not Saddam Hussein should have been removed from power, or whether toppling his regime was in the best national interests of the United States or other nations, let alone the Iraqi people. This is a discussion of the evidence put forth by the Bush administration to justify the invasion.

Over the strong objections of Vice President Dick Cheney, who thought that President Bush had the authority to invade without consulting either congress or the United Nations—George W. Bush sought the approval of both. Ultimately, he also made his case directly to the American people. It was a case based on distinct and specific pieces of evidence that were woven together into a compelling argument that Saddam Hussein had stockpiles of weapons of mass destruction (WMD) and that he was actively seeking nuclear weapons. This was in flagrant violation of at least two United Nations resolutions.

In keeping with the theme of this book, our analysis should center on how information is processed through filters that alter the fraction of what is observed versus the totality of available evidence. Previous chapters have introduced confirmation bias and cherry-picking as processes that distort our perception of the world by selectively noticing, focusing on, and evaluating evidence through a filter of preexisting beliefs or agendas. For the fraction (evidence that supports your belief/all evidence), the error—as we have established—is focusing on the numerator and ignoring the denominator. Because the arguments the Bush administration put forth to justify invasion of Iraq were evidence-based arguments, how biases and distortions of evidence alter conclusions is of great relevance to this story. After all, what could be more consequential than the decision to go to war?

It was a reasonable suspicion that Saddam Hussein had WMD and a reasonable assumption that he was eager to make more and was willing to use them. In violation of the Geneva Convention, he had used chemical weapons in his war with Iran and also on his own people. Chemical and biological weapons had been found in Iraq after the First Gulf War, and his previous attempts to generate weapons-grade uranium were uncontested. Moreover, after the First Gulf War, the Iraqi government clearly lied to inspectors for the United Nations Special Commission (UNSCOM) multiple times, continually modifying their weapons declarations, preventing or evading inspections, and failing to document the destruction of the amount of chemical and biological weapons they previously catalogued as having in their possession. Then, in 1997, Iraq expelled weapons inspectors altogether.

In response, the United States and United Kingdom launched a four-day bombing campaign in 1998 with the goal of hobbling Iraq's ability to produce WMD. In 2003, inspectors had not been allowed back into Iraq since they had been expelled, and intelligence agencies had a hard time recruiting spies within Iraq who could provide information. So, Iraq was an opaque box that neither the United Nations nor the United States could see into, other than with aerial photographs.

Given Saddam Hussein's previous activities of WMD production and his willingness to use them, his evasive efforts to avoid inspections, his failure to account for weapons he was known to previously have, and the lack of inspections for several years, it was a reasonable supposition that he had WMD. This was still an inference, however. What was the actual evidence?

To make the case for invasion, the Bush administration presented a cadre of damning evidence to the U.S. Congress, to the United Nations, and to the American people. Much of this evidence came from a National Intelligence Estimate (NIE), which is a document that synthesizes the consensus view of multiple intelligence agencies. Additional information came from other sources. In aggregate, it added up to what seemed like a compelling case—a case that the Bush administration put forward with great confidence, both in private and public forums. Both President Bush and then–Secretary of State Colin Powell spoke directly to the United Nations, and President Bush gave a State of the Union address to a joint session of Congress. Overall, a series of specific claims were made, including the following:

1. Iraq had chemical weapons. No direct evidence indicated that such was the case, but one could infer this was true based on past activities, aerial photos of buildings and trucks that could be chemical plants, and the lack of any inspections.

2. It was considered highly likely that Iraq had biological weapons. Iraq had them before, and almost certainly, they had them again—or had never destroyed them in the first place. In his speech to the United Nations, Powell referred to intelligence from within Iraq, based on eyewitness testimony of an Iraqi, that they had mobile biological weapons factories on trucks that could move around to avoid detection. Such trucks could easily produce batches of potent biological weapons in an overnight fermentation. Powell even showed the United Nations an image of what one would look like and how it would work.

3. With regards to nuclear weapons, Saddam Hussein was stated to be working in a deal to purchase large quantities of radioactive material (i.e., yellowcake) from Niger, which he could refine into fissile material. Iraq also was known to have purchased highly suspect aluminum tubes, which were determined to be suitable as centrifuge tubes to refine the yellowcake.

4. Iraq was determined to be developing unmanned aerial vehicles (UAVs) that could be shipped to the coast of the United States, could be flown over American cities, and then could spray chemical or biological weapons on highly populated areas. Of high concern, an Iraqi agent had attempted to purchase global positioning satellite (GPS) devices with maps of American cities programmed into them.

5. In addition to all of these problems, Iraq had close relationships with Al Qaeda, linking them both to previous attacks (such as the attack on the World Trade Center on September 11, 2001) and also making them more dangerous with regard to future attacks.

The NIE was highly speculative, and those who prepared it were clearly aware of this. For example, it stated, "Although we have little specific information on Iraq's chemical weapons stockpile, Saddam probably has stocked at least 100 metric tons and possibly as much as 500 metric tons of chemical weapons agents—much of it added in the last year." Clearly, it was an educated guess based on "little specific information." Years later, in an interview, former Secretary of Defense Donald Rumsfeld made the comment: "If it were a fact, it wouldn't be called intelligence."[1] In other words, none of it was direct proof. This was not like the photographs of Soviet missiles in Cuba in 1962, which President Kennedy used as evidence during the Cuban Missile Crisis. Rather, the evidence regarding Iraq was indirect. Of course, intelligence is almost always at least somewhat speculative; the Cuban missile photos were exceptional. The uncertain nature of intelligence information, however, was not conveyed to the public; rather, the Bush administration presented the evidence regarding WMD in Iraq as established facts.

Despite a lack of any actual direct evidence, in a public speech in August 2002 to the Veterans of Foreign Wars, Cheney said, "Simply stated, there is no doubt that Saddam Hussein now has weapons of mass destruction; there is no doubt that he is amassing them to use against our friends, against our allies, and against us."[2] It's unclear how assessments based on "little specific information" in the NIE equated to "no doubt"; but this is the rhetoric that was being put forth. The same level of confidence was being expressed in smaller settings by other administration officials. In the summer of 2002, a subordinate of Paul Wolfowitz (then undersecretary of defense) was quoted as telling a group of guests at the American embassy in Egypt, "Saddam has nuclear weapons." When the American ambassador asked if this was based on an assessment by American intelligence, the response was "we don't need one . . . we already know it."[3]

On September 12, 2002, President Bush addressed the United Nations specifically requesting a new resolution, which the United Nations Security Council unanimously passed on November 8 (Resolution 1441). The new resolution gave Iraq 30 days to provide "a currently accurate, full, and complete declaration of all aspects of its programmes to develop chemical, biological, and nuclear weapons," as well as to give UN inspectors "immediate, unimpeded, unconditional, and unrestricted access" to all facilities.

By all accounts, Iraq complied with this new resolution. Before any inspections took place, in a speech to the Cincinnati Museum Center in October 2002, President Bush declared, "Surveillance photos reveal that the regime is rebuilding facilities that it had used to produce chemical and biological weapons," that "Saddam Hussein still has chemical and biological weapons and is increasing his capabilities to make more. And he is moving ever closer to developing a nuclear weapon," that "Iraq has attempted to purchase high-strength aluminum tubes and other equipment needed for gas centrifuges, which are used to enrich uranium for nuclear weapons," and that "We've learned that Iraq has trained al Qaeda members in bomb-making and poisons and deadly gases."[4]

In compliance with Resolution 1441, by November 27, Iraq allowed inspectors to enter the country and submitted a long declaration of weapons, but the declaration basically had nothing new in it. This meant one of two things: either they had not reconstituted their weapons program, or they were lying. In the latter case, this would serve as the justification for invasion, at least as per the UN resolution. Demonstrating that Iraq did indeed have WMD and was failing to declare them became the focus of the Bush administration.[5] After several months of work, however, the UN inspection teams had failed to find any evidence of WMD, but they were continuing on with their efforts.

On January 28, 2003, in his State of the Union address to a joint session of congress, President Bush stated, "The British government has learned that Saddam Hussein recently sought significant quantities of uranium from Africa." Then, on February 5, 2003, Powell addressed the United Nations regarding Iraq's violation of UN Resolution 1441. Powell was, at that time, likely the most publicly credible and trustworthy member of the Bush administration, more so than even President Bush. Powell's credibility was based on a lifetime of service to his nation, in and out of uniform, through which he repeatedly showed honesty and integrity, both in word and deed. His presentation was reminiscent of when Adlai Stevenson addressed the United Nations during the Cuban Missile Crisis, at which time Stevenson presented photographs of Soviet missiles installed in Cuba, tantamount to proof of what the U.S.S.R. had been denying. In contrast, the evidence presented by Powell was far less direct, was far less compelling, and ultimately was being used to argue for, not against, direct military conflict.

Powell's presentation focused on Iraq's refusal to declare and allow inspections of biological weapons, chemical weapons, and materials needed to assemble nuclear weapons. Assertions were made that Iraq had, was continuing to make, and was hiding WMD from inspection teams. Powell showed aerial surveillance photos suggesting that Iraqis had notice of when inspectors would arrive at certain sites and were able to move contraband material to avoid detection. Powell played audiotapes of intercepted phone calls suggesting that Iraqis knew in advance when inspectors were coming and were removing incriminating evidence. Powell referred to the aluminum tubes for uranium enrichment, stating that "all the experts who have analyzed the tubes in our possession agree that they can be adapted for centrifuge use."

Although Powell chose his words carefully and expressed some amount of circumspection, the language was nevertheless presented largely in factual terms. In his words:

> Indeed, the facts and Iraq's behavior show that Saddam Hussein and his regime are concealing their efforts to produce more weapons of mass destruction. . . . These are not assertions. What we're giving you are facts and conclusions based on solid intelligence. . . . Ladies and gentlemen, these are not assertions. These are facts, corroborated by many sources, some of them sources of the intelligence services of other countries.[6]

On March 19, 2003, just six weeks later, the United States (along with the United Kingdom and other allies) invaded Iraq under the justification that Iraq had failed to comply with UN Resolution 1441 to disclose its WMD. But Iraq allowed inspections and the inspectors had found nothing, so how had they failed to comply? Of course, the inspections were not done yet; perhaps the weapons were there but the inspectors had just not found them so far. Although UN inspections had made good progress up to this point, and their director, Hans Blix, assured the United Nations that completion of the inspections would take only a few more months, the United States was unwilling to wait. The position of the Bush administration was that Iraq must be hiding the weapons. President Bush and his allies were going in with force and were going to find the weapons and seize them, as well as remove Saddam Hussein's regime from power. Enough was enough. The sentiments were well reflected in a phrase often repeated by the Bush administration, first coined by National Security Adviser Condoleezza Rice, "We don't want the smoking gun to be a mushroom cloud."[7]

As military advisers had predicted, the Iraqi army was rapidly defeated. Month after month went by during the occupation that followed, and no WMD were found. Ultimately, it was determined that, indeed, Iraq had not declared any WMD because they did not have any. The reason the inspectors didn't find any WMD was because they did not exist. At this point, the question was asked, "what went wrong"? Of course, it is not necessarily the case that anything went wrong. Sometimes rational and balanced evaluation of evidence leads to an incorrect result—we live in a world of uncertainty. A detailed analysis of how evidence was collected, interpreted, and presented seemed necessary, however, particularly given the outcome.

Quantity and Quality of the Evidence in the Context of All the Evidence

On September 12, the same day Bush was addressing the United Nations to ask for a new resolution, the dialog with the Congress was already heating up. Senator Dick Durbin was frustrated that Congress had not been provided with an NIE. Indeed, no effort to produce an NIE had even been underway. Durbin basically demanded that an NIE be assembled and presented to Congress, as was customary, especially when matters of grave concern were under consideration. Indeed, the NIE that was subsequently presented to Congress served as the basis for the majority of the five major claims listed earlier.

Typically, an NIE takes at least several months to prepare, sometimes as much as a year; however, Congress was set to vote on whether or not to authorize the president to invade Iraq, and Durbin demanded an NIE no later than October 1, in just nineteen days. Consensus for an NIE can be hard to reach even under optimal circumstances, and it requires careful dialog and vetting of information among agencies—with only nineteen days, this could be nothing more than a rush job. As one of the producers of the NIE would later say in an interview with Robert Draper, "We had to do the best we could. The problem was, the best we could do sucked."[8]

In his landmark book on the topic *To Start a War*, Robert Draper analyzed this process, including detailed interviews with a number of the intelligence agents involved. Intelligence agencies, and the CIA in particular, were under tremendous pressure to provide evidence that supported the claims that the Bush administration wanted to make. That, however, is not what intelligence agencies do, or at least not what they are supposed to do. Intelligence agencies are supposed to give the best analysis of a situation that they can, based on whatever evidence they can get, and with careful evaluation of the quality of the evidence. As one intelligence official involved with the process reflected, "The first thing they teach you in CIA 101 is you don't help them make the case. . . . But we were all infected in the case for war."[9]

A famous (or perhaps infamous) conversation took place between President Bush and George Tenet (then director of the CIA) on December 21, 2002, a month before Bush's State of the Union address. The White House had requested the CIA to put together a succinct presentation to build the case for invading Iraq, a presentation that could be used to convince the public. The evidence that they had was so unpersuasive that President Bush's response was simply, "Nice try." Bush followed his request by stating: "Look, in about five weeks I may have to ask the fathers and mothers of America to send their sons and daughters off to war. This has to be well developed. We have to be aware of the need to sell this to the average citizen. So, it needs to be more convincing. Probably needs some better examples." This put the CIA in a difficult position. What better examples? They had already used the best evidence they had. At this point, the president turned to Tenet and said, "Can you do this George?" Tenet replied, "Slam dunk."[10]

One year later, when no WMD had been found, Bush specifically referenced this moment to blame the CIA for getting it wrong.[11] Bush was listening to his own intelligence agencies and acting on what they had told him was a sure thing, a "slam dunk." However, as George Tenet explained in an interview on *60 Minutes* and later in his book *At the Center of the Storm*,[12] the "slam dunk" comment was in response to the question: "Can you frame the existing evidence in a way that makes it compelling to the American people?" and not "Are you yourself convinced of the case?"[13] The idea that the CIA was entirely confident in its intelligence and the president was acting on their recommendation is, by all accounts, revisionist history that allowed Bush to throw the CIA under the bus, rather than acknowledge his mistake.

Sadly, numerous analyses published by different experts have reviewed the arguments that the Bush administration made, years after the fact, and shown clear selective assessment of information. They focused on the molehills of data that supported a conclusion of WMDs and ignored mountains of evidence to the contrary. It is not possible to tell from this pattern of behavior whether it was an intentional act (e.g., cherry-picking) or subconscious (e.g., confirmation bias), but the two are by no means mutually exclusive.

In Jeffrey Jay Matthew's biography of Colin Powell, it is written that "Powell and other government leaders suffered from a classic—indeed catastrophic-case of 'confirmation bias,' whereby they largely dismissed information in the National Intelligence Estimate that conflicted with what they believed to be true about Iraq and amplified information that seemed to confirm their dire and erroneous beliefs." In Powell's own words, "you really, really have to bore down far more deeply than we did at that time with respect to the intelligence."[14] Given the complex mixture of people in the Bush administration, it was almost certainly a combination of confirmation bias and cherry-picking. Making the distinction requires an understanding of the source of the preexisting beliefs, and the personalities and motivations involved.

Background Beliefs, Motivations, and Agendas in the Bush Administration

Although the ultimate decision to invade Iraq was President Bush's alone, the process was the product of an entire administration. While the president's mind is a single cognition, the president's administration consists of multiple personalities, multiple perspectives, and multiple priorities all simultaneously at play. How such networks of players may affect belief is an important issue; however, for the current discussion, it is worth examining each player individually. Confirmation bias and cherry-picking depend on the background beliefs and agendas of the individuals involved.

Cheney and Rumsfeld, as well as many of their staff, seem to have been eager to invade Iraq for quite some time, in many cases long before September 11, 2001, and with supreme confidence in the ease of their victory and a triumphant outcome. Rice was likely far more conflicted, and was no great friend of either Cheney or Rumsfeld; however, she had grand ambitions of democratizing the Middle East. Powell was strongly against invasion, not because he was any great fan of Saddam Hussein and not because he thought the invasion would fail. Rather, Powell fully understood the implications of being responsible for the entire situation once invasion was complete, with no easy way out.

As for the president, it seemed to be a combination of the strength of conviction that it was America's role to bring freedom to the rest of the world as well as a strong evangelical sense of righteousness. The Bush family also likely had a vendetta because Saddam Hussein apparently had made an attempt to assassinate George H. W. Bush (Bush Senior).[15] In addition, the president's personal wealth had strong ties to the oil industry, as did the vice president's, who was the former CEO of Halliburton and was still holding deferred stock options from the company.[16] Moreover, as warned about by President Eisenhower in his farewell address, the military industrial complex gets rich when America goes to war, and immense sums of money are spent on lobbying politicians.

More idealistically, the Bush administration felt that replacing Saddam Hussein with a friendlier and more benevolent government would be both strategically important to the United States and also a great benefit to the Middle East. Setting aside how likely this really was to occur, it would be a great strategic move for America. Finally, in politics, the name of the game is staying in the game—politicians are never that far away from the next election. The United States had received a horrible wound from the September 11 attacks, and lashing out at enemies appealed to many voters at a deep emotional level.

For all of these reasons, one may believe the United States should have, or should not have, invaded Iraq; however, none of these are the reasons given by the Bush administration. Rather, these were the sources of preconceived beliefs. The actual reasons presented were twofold. The first (as just described) was that Saddam Hussein had WMD in violation of UN Resolution 1441 and that this was an intolerable risk to the United States and the world. The second, which was oddly built into the narrative, but was not part of the UN resolution, was that Iraq was responsible for the September 11 attacks.

Linking Saddam Hussein to Osama bin Laden and Iraq to Al Qaeda

To understand the full narrative, one has to go back to the attack on the World Trade Center, but not the attack that took place on September 11, 2001. Rather, this story begins with the 1993 bombing of the World Trade Center, in which a truck full of explosives was detonated in the parking garage beneath the building. Although this did not threaten the structural integrity of the building, it did substantial damage and injured 1,000 people (killing six of them). Ultimately, seven conspirators were arrested, convicted, and sentenced to prison—they were mostly Pakistani or Egyptian nationals with radical ideologies focused on attacking the United States in defense of the plight of the Palestinian people.

At that time, and subsequently, the theory was put forth that Iraq had supported the terrorists who carried out the bombing. Multiple intelligence agencies, including the CIA, however, dismissed this theory as invalid. Nevertheless, a number of people vociferously supported this idea—perhaps none more so than Laurie Mylroie, a Harvard professor who published a book entitled *Study of Revenge: Saddam Hussein's Unfinished War Against America*.[17]

What was the evidence that linked Saddam Hussein to the 1993 attack? Of the seven individuals involved, one (and only one) was of Iraqi descent, although he was born in the United States. In addition, when looking through all the cell phone records of the other perpetrators (including hundreds of calls), one of them (who was not himself of Iraqi decent), had placed 46 calls to his uncle, who had been a Palestinian terrorist, and was now living in Iraq. These 46 calls were placed over an eight-month period of time, and their contents are unknown. That was the link, that was the evidence, pretty much all of it. Essentially every credible intelligence analysis dismissed this idea, as did most analyses by political scientists. The unsupported idea that Iraq was somehow behind the attack, however, made a big impression on Paul Wolfowitz.

Wolfowitz had been the undersecretary of defense under Bush Senior and was frustrated that Saddam Hussein had been left in power after operation Desert Storm (i.e., the First Gulf War that had forced Saddam Hussein out of Kuwait, which he previously had invaded). Wolfowitz deeply regretted, and carried much personal guilt, for how the United States had encouraged an uprising by the Iraqi people and had then failed to support them, allowing the uprising to be crushed by Saddam Hussein's forces. Mylroie clearly had the strong belief that Saddam Hussein was attacking the United States and was interpreting information through that filter. For example, she even went so far as to argue that Saddam Hussein had been behind the Oklahoma City bombings in 1995. Wolfowitz did not accept this latter argument as it was too far-fetched even for him; however, he swallowed the connection between Hussein and the 1993 World Trade Center bombing, hook, line, and sinker.

Wolfowitz consistently attempted to draw connections between Iraq and attacks on the United States. For example, in 1998, Wolfowitz (along with Rumsfeld with whom he was serving on a commission) specifically requested the CIA to try to link Iraq to the 1993 bombing, but the CIA found no such link. Wolfowitz was undeterred by such expert analyses and dedicated much of his time to an unrelenting effort to inspire strategies to unseat Saddam Hussein, authoring a piece in the *Weekly Standard* (along with Zalmay M. Khalilzad) titled "Overthrow Him."[18]

In early 2001, Wolfowitz found himself once again serving in a presidential administration, as the deputy secretary of defense under Rumsfeld, who reported directly to President Bush. Continuing with his agenda, he had both the CIA and FBI reinvestigate Laurie Mylroie's claims of a link between the 1993 World Trade Center bombing and Saddam Hussein. Again, the answer was there was no actual connection. He continued his efforts in this regard, as well as formulating theoretical plans to overthrow Saddam Hussein. These plans consisted of seizing the oil fields in southern Iraq with the goal of inspiring an uprising of Iraqi nationals who would then take over the country—essentially a "do over" of the failed uprising at the end of the First Gulf War. Of course, the notion of seizing the oil fields did not hurt in appealing to the corporate interests who would benefit from such a maneuver.

Wolfowitz consistently hit barriers with his plans and arguments, until the entire political atmosphere changed on September 11, 2001. He immediately attempted to implicate Iraq and Saddam Hussein in the September 11 attacks, citing evidence that Iraqi intelligence agents had met with Osama bin Laden in 1995 and formed a relationship. The CIA, however, had detailed intelligence that in the 1995 meeting, Al Qaeda had specifically rejected a partnership with Iraq. All intelligence pointed to Al Qaeda being independently responsible and that their efforts were facilitated by the Taliban in Afghanistan, not by Saddam Hussein in Iraq. Operation Enduring Freedom was launched and the U.S. military attacked Al Qaeda in Afghanistan, but it stopped with Afghanistan, at least initially.

Through a strategic combination of U.S. Special Forces, advanced air power, and collaboration with Afghani opposition forces, the Taliban was driven out of power and a secular government replaced it. Osama bin Laden escaped, but Al Qaeda was defeated and dispersed. During this process, U.S. intelligence acquired large amounts of Al Qaeda records and documents, which showed stunning progress on generating and gaining access to advanced biological, chemical, and nuclear weapons. They had thankfully not done so, but they were much further along than anyone had thought when Operation Enduring Freedom had been launched. Contrary to the link to Iraq that Wolfowitz was pushing, not a single seized document from the entire cache indicated any dialog or relationship between Iraq and Al Qaeda. This highly pertinent "negative data" was of little use to Wolfowitz, as it did not confirm his preexisting belief. Rather, he chose to focus on a single solitary piece of evidence obtained from a senior Al Qaeda agent (Ibn al-Shaykh al-Libi).

al-Libi stated that, in 2000, two Al Qaeda members had gone to Baghdad to learn how to generate and use chemical and biological weapons, and Wolfowitz pointed to this evidence as proof that Iraq was sponsoring Al Qaeda attacks. Wolfowitz was cherry-picking the single bit of information that supported his theory and ignoring the lack of any other information despite the great volumes of correspondence that had been captured. The lives of his fellow citizens were at stake: given the gravity of another terrorist attack, wasn't it prudent to focus on evidence even if it was not substantial evidence? This might be a reasonable point of view; after all, wasn't the failure to prevent the September 11 attack an error in not paying attention to small bits of evidence, ignoring the proverbial needle in a haystack?

Of course, the smaller the amount of evidence available, the more important its quality becomes. If this single piece of evidence was going to inform policy, shouldn't one make sure it was reliable evidence? How confident were intelligence agencies in al-Libi's statement, under what circumstances had it been obtained, and had it been verified by other sources?

al-Libi had not mentioned anything about Iraq, even after withstanding days of "enhanced interrogation techniques" by U.S. agents. Rather, only after the Americans handed him over to Egyptian interrogators did al-Libi finally state this "fact" under unknown circumstances of interrogation. Even the CIA was highly skeptical of this information, later dismissing it as a fabrication resulting from torture, which is known to produce unreliable intelligence. After some point, people will say anything their interrogators want them to say to stop their own suffering. Ultimately, the CIA officially disavowed the accuracy of this information, but not until after the United States invaded Iraq.[19] As explained next, given how the Bush administration handled evidence, it is not clear that the CIA disavowing the information would have made any difference.

The potential link between Iraq and Al Qaeda became ever more important on September 11, 2001. Wolfowitz, along with Scooter Libby (Dick Cheney's chief of staff), hounded the CIA regarding a possible link of the September 11 hijackers to Iraq. Not a single one of the nineteen hijackers was an Iraqi national (most were from Saudi Arabia). Czech diplomats did report that Mohamed Atta, who had hijacked American Airlines Flight 11 (along with four others), had met with an Iraqi intelligence officer at the Iraqi embassy in Prague in April 2001. A careful analysis of this information by the CIA revealed that it was thin, at best. Atta had been in the United States before and after the alleged meeting, and there was no record of him flying to Europe. Of course, he could have flown there and back under an alias. The Czech report, however, was based on an anonymous informant who had identified Atta from a newspaper photo—and even based on these questionable circumstances, the informant was only "70 percent sure."

Wolfowitz kept asking the same question over and over again: Was there a link between Iraq and Al Qaeda? He kept getting the same answer, "no," which he found unacceptable, earning him a description by one CIA analyst as an "obsessive fanatic." Wolfowitz was not alone. Vice President Chaney, and some of his aides, also pursued the Atta meeting with great vigor, tasking a full paper from the CIA on the question.

Tenet oversaw the writing of this paper, which presented the single piece of evidence suggesting the meeting occurred (e.g., the anonymous source who was 70 percent sure based on a newspaper photo) against multiple other pieces of data suggesting the meeting never took place. In addition, the CIA was analyzing the event in a broader context. Saddam Hussein was a secular leader, one who had many enemies in religious groups that wanted him ousted; his close collaboration with an Islamic extremist organization like Al Qaeda was not a natural fit. Still, with a mutual hatred of the United States as a unifying factor, one had to consider the possibility, and consider it carefully. Indeed, the CIA did this, as is their job, but they still did not find a connection. Despite this deep skepticism in the formal assessment by the CIA, Cheney stated on national television that the meeting with Atta was "pretty well confirmed."[20]

Being unable to coerce or push the CIA into supporting the idea of a relationship between Iraq and Al Qaeda, the White House then tasked a different intelligence group at the Department of Defense to find a connection. In the words of a CIA analyst, "They were taking raw traffic completely out of context . . . simply with the determination to make the case," and adding, "They were connecting dots that weren't even there . . . It was one percent. It was moons away. It was six degrees of Kevin Bacon's mom."[21]

The CIA produced its own analysis, entirely discrediting the conclusions of the Department of Defense group—the CIA's analysis was entirely dismissed. Facing the prospect of becoming irrelevant and being shut out of the process entirely, the CIA director ultimately acquiesced to give a report to Congress that supported a link between Iraq and Al Qaeda. Regrettably, the link between Iraq and Al Qaeda just did not hold water, despite Wolfowitz and others forcing the CIA into complicity through attrition. Nevertheless, this was the evidence to support the fifth claim listed at the beginning of this chapter—pretty much the only evidence, in fact. Given all of the data that was in the administration's possession, this is an extreme case of cherry-picking, as the highly pertinent negative findings were simply ignored (e.g., no actual correspondence between Al Qaeda and Iraq found in the large number of documents seized).

The lack of credible evidence ultimately did not matter. A significant percentage of Americans already believed Saddam Hussein was responsible for the September 11 attacks. By six months after September 11, President Bush had basically ceased making statements mentioning Osama bin Laden in favor of making statements about Saddam Hussein at the same time he was banging the drum of the War on Terror, likely reinforcing what Americans were predisposed to believe (figure 6.1).[22]

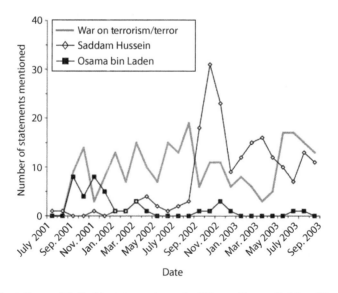

6.1 President George W. Bush's statements on the War on Terror, Saddam Hussein, and Osama bin Laden, month by month.

Source: From Scott L. Althaus and Devon M. Largio, *When Osama Became Saddam: Origins and Consequences of the Change in America's Public Enemy #1* (Cambridge: Cambridge University Press, 2004). Reprinted with permission of Cambridge University Press.

The Tenuous Nature of the Other Claims of Fact

So, the link between Iraq and Al Qaeda was tenuous at best but was presented as fact and many Americans accepted it. What about the rest of the evidence that was used to justify invasion? To be fair, everyone in the intelligence community and the White House was legitimately on high alert. This process went all the way up to President Bush who was receiving a "daily threat matrix" from the FBI that contained raw unprocessed intelligence that had not undergone scrutiny or verification. As stated by Rice in an interview with Robert Draper, "If some nutcase was going to blow up Sears Tower from a phone booth in Minnesota, it was on the president's desk."[23]

This situation was quite natural. The September 11 attacks had not been prevented because minute warning signs had not been noticed. Then, shortly after September 11, live anthrax spores had been mailed to a number of people, resulting in illness and several deaths—terror was ongoing and everyone was concerned. So, in the zeal to avoid a second attack, sensitivity to even trace information was very high. When this happens, small pieces of data can become extreme; confirmation bias is amplified in this setting. The combination of such bias with others who have a specific agenda and are purposefully cherry-picking data can be an overwhelming force.

So, what about the actual basis for the other assertions of the five facts listed at the beginning of this chapter regarding chemical weapons, mobile biological weapons factories, yellowcake and aluminum tubes to refine uranium, and UAVs to poison American cities? What about evading the inspectors, moving contraband material from warehouses just before UN inspectors arrived, and always staying a step ahead?

The basis for assuming chemical weapons was always inferential, based on past behavior and poor documentation of how previous weapons were disposed of. As for newly manufactured capacities, Iraq did have plants to generate chemicals, but all of these had highly legitimate uses for everyday industrial purposes, and they would be found in any industrial society. Indeed, the Bush administration noted this specifically, claiming that Iraq had purposefully woven its chemical weapons production capabilities into legitimate factories, making weapon production impossible to detect. This was a classic tautology; the absence of any evidence of chemical weapons was proof of a great conspiracy to hide chemical weapons production. Indeed, we know it was a truly excellent conspiracy, for only an expert conspiracy would leave no evidence. Evidence of weapons would be nice, but lack of evidence is the strongest proof because it confirms they must be hiding something; otherwise, we would have found it because we *know* it is there.

Why couldn't the Iraqis really have been hiding their weapons? They had done so before. Wasn't it fair to assume they were doing so now? What about

Iraqis finding out where inspectors were going and moving contraband just before they arrived, as was demonstrated by Powell in his UN speech? One of the inspectors from the very photo that Powell showed commented: "I'm in that photo . . . I went into that bunker that those trucks pulled up to. There was a three-inch layer of pigeon dung covering everything. And a layer of dust on top of that. There's no way someone came in and cleaned that place out. No way they could've faked that."[24]

What about the basis for believing that Iraq had mobile biological chemical factories? The evidence for this came from the testimony from an Iraqi chemical engineer, Rafid Ahmed Alwan al-Janabi, who had arrived in Germany in 1999 seeking asylum. U.S. intelligence agencies could not find evidence of biological weapons factories from their satellite images, but why not? The information from al-Janabi solved the problem perfectly: they couldn't find the factories because they were moving around—ingenious. German intelligence agencies, however, rapidly determined that al-Janabi was not a credible witness. His testimony did not line up with that of others. His description of the mobile factories, however, did line up perfectly with what UN inspectors had speculated about in their final report. In fact, it lined up so perfectly that German intelligence agencies suspected al-Janabi had simply copied the details of those reports, which were publicly available on the internet.[25]

Why would al-Janabi lie? It may have helped him stay in Germany, including an income, a Mercedes, and an apartment. It is more likely, however, that he hated Saddam Hussein's regime and wanted to bring it down. How do we know this? Al-Janabi admitted it outright in an interview with *The Guardian* newspaper in 2011.[26]

The basis for Saddam Hussein's seeking nuclear weapons was on even weaker footing. It is true that an intelligence report had come to the United States from Italian intelligence services in early 2002 reporting that Iraq had convinced Niger to sell 500 tons of yellowcake (a source of uranium) to Iraq per year. According to an internal memo that was subsequently declassified, U.S. intelligence analysts rapidly determined that the report was unlikely to be true, because of political and economic issues, as well as the difficulty in transporting the yellowcake.[27] Nevertheless, out of due diligence, the former U.S. ambassador to Niger (Joseph C. Wilson) was sent to Niger to investigate, as was four-star General Carlton W. Fulford Jr. Neither Ambassador Wilson nor General Fulford were impressed with what they found, and both seriously doubted the report.

With regards to the aluminum centrifuge tubes, without doubt, Iraq had purchased them, as they were physically seized en route to Iraq. Moreover, the CIA reported that its analysts agreed that they were intended to enrich uranium. Internal analysts disagreed widely, however, on whether or not these tubes could be used for uranium enrichment, as did experts at the department of energy, many of whom felt the tubes did not have the physical properties for such purposes.[28] Still, some felt they might be used for that purpose, and some also thought that other items purchased by Iraq could have been used in centrifuges (e.g., certain magnets). This conclusion might have been correct; however, in this case, the strength of the evidence and the consensus on its quality was exaggerated when it was included in the NIE with confidence. Some dissenting opinions were included in the report, but only in a footnote.[29]

Finally, the claim that the GPS devices that contained maps of U.S. cities and the assumption that they would be used to guide UAVs that would spray toxins or biological weapons on America were not as farfetched as they may sound. Saddam Hussein had a well-known UAV program, and it was documented that his plan was to use UAVs to spray biological toxins on unsuspecting people. According to an interview by Draper with a senior Bush adviser, this in particular really worried President Bush and motivated his thinking. It was exactly the type of nightmare scenario he was determined not to let happen again on his watch.[30]

The CIA did question the Iraqi who attempted to buy the GPS devices. He claimed that the devices would not work without the mapping software, as the manufacturer clearly described. This was the only reason he included it in the order, but it seems fair for intelligence analysts to have been skeptical about that claim.

Reflecting Back on the Run Up to Invasion of Iraq

It is all too easy to analyze an uncertain event, in retrospect, with the benefit of knowing the outcome and the wisdom of hindsight. This is what Cheney referred to as "Monday Morning Quarterbacking" in a 2011 interview with Wolf Blitzer in which Cheney defended his statements from before the war that "There was no doubt" about Saddam Hussein having WMD. Acknowledging that weapons were never found, he reflected that "there was no doubt at the time."[31] He argued that a reasonable determination was made with the information available to them. That there was no doubt reflects only on how confident he remembers himself and the administration being and not on how strong the actual evidence was.

Ironically, reassessing information after the fact is itself a form of confirmation bias. One is interpreting data from a previous time, when the outcome was not known. But now it is known, and we cannot unknow it. This is often called hindsight bias. One of the problems of confirmation bias is that it always attaches to whatever beliefs we hold, even to true ones. This affects how we judge how others weighed the evidence, but they did not know then what we know now. In other words, the previous arguments seem weaker to us now than they did to the people involved at the time the arguments were being made. This is the case not only because we do not have the confirmation bias they had back then but also because we have our new hindsight bias now, driven by our current belief that Iraq had no WMD.

Politics is a dirty business, with all manner of conflicting interests, motivators, and factors at play. In addition to confirmation bias, purposeful, aggressive, and vicious cherry-picking was almost certainly going on as well. When Ambassador Wilson returned from Niger and reported that Niger was not selling yellowcake to Iraq, and printed an editorial about it, retribution seemed to be swift. A senior Bush administration official mentioned to a journalist that Wilson's wife, Valerie Plame was a covert CIA operative—a fact that the journalist then published, ending Plame's intelligence career, and potentially endangering her life. It has been reported that multiple members of the Bush administration leaked this information in retribution for Wilson's report.[32] Valerie Plame specifically named Scooter Libby as being the source of the leak.[33] The journalist who reported Valerie Plame's identity as a CIA operative confirmed that he did learn it from a senior administration official, but he claims that it was an offhand remark—this remark nevertheless was confirmed by an independent official.[34]

A formal determination of who leaked the information was never made. Libby, however, was convicted of obstruction of justice and perjury in the investigation of the leak. His 30-month sentence was never served, being commuted by President Bush, and he was subsequently pardoned by President Trump. Although we do not really know precisely what happened, a key witness against Libby did recant her testimony and Libby's law license was reinstated.[35] It seems pretty unlikely that the leak was accidental, however, whether by Libby or someone else.

Moreover, the Bush administration had a regrettable pattern of exacting retribution upon those who voiced dissent. Before the Iraq War, General Eric Shinseki was the chief of staff of the army and a member of the joint chiefs of staff. In public testimony, he estimated that far more troops would be required than the Bush administration was proposing, if Iraq was invaded. After making the assessment, General Shinseki was rapidly attacked by both Rumsfeld and Wolfowitz and was professionally marginalized as a punishment for his disagreement.[36] Kori Schake, the director for defense strategy from 2002 to 2005, pointed out that "it served to silence critics just at the point in time when, internal to the process, you most wanted critical judgement."[37] Regrettably, General Shinseki turned out to be entirely correct.

One can hardly imagine that intelligence operatives do not fear reprisal for reporting things the government does not want to hear. This fact has been confirmed by many of the interviews carried out by Robert Draper with CIA officers directly involved with the pre-war assessment of Iraq's WMD.[38] Although we cannot specifically know what was in the minds of the Bush administration, we at least understand their behavior. Such behavior is by no means particular to the Bush administration. Almost identical patterns were seen before Bush (in the Nixon administration) and after Bush in the Trump administration. The threat of such retribution is likely ubiquitous at some level, both inside and outside of politics. It may or may not be good politics, but it is certainly not good for human perception and reasoning.

Lest one think I am picking on Republicans, the Vietnam conflict was generated and perpetuated mostly under Democratic administrations. A careful analysis of both the confirmation bias surrounding Vietnam, and outright lies told to the American people, demonstrate errors as egregious, if not more so, than the run up to the Iraq War.

More recently, reporting of causalities during President Obama's administration revealed an instance in which modifying a fraction resulted in substantial public misinformation. In 2012, the Obama administration reported a substantial decrease in attacks referred to as "enemy-initiated attacks." The decrease in this metric was presented as clear evidence that the United States was making significant military progress in Afghanistan.

In 2012, Afghan soldiers were doing more and more of the fighting and U.S. soldiers were doing less of it. As more Afghan and fewer U.S. soldiers were fighting, enemy-initiated attacks increased on Afghan soldiers and decreased on U.S. troops, even though the number of attacks overall was the same. Although U.S. and allied Afghan troops were fighting together, only attacks on U.S. troops were counted as an "enemy-initiated attack."[39] So, the reported number of attacks went down, when in fact the actual number of attacks was unaltered. If your concern was just the safety of U.S. troops, then this is a perfectly reasonable metric. As an indication that progress was being made in the war, however, the metric was highly misleading. The Obama administration subsequently acknowledged this issue and claimed that it was a clerical error. Whether intentional or accidental, this is yet another example of a distortion of meaning through misrepresenting a fraction.[40]

Summary

In this chapter, we explored, in detail, one particular instance of how confirmation bias and cherry-picking data can affect governments going to war. The Iraq War was analyzed because data and evidence were the basis the government put forward to justify war. Because of the hard work of journalists and historians, we now have considerable information about the administration's thinking and how it was shaped.

The role of confirmation bias and cherry-picking is a persistent problem regarding decisions by nations to go to war. In her book *The March of Folly: From Troy to Vietnam*, the historian and author Barbara W. Tuchman chronicles, in astounding and terrifying detail, how confirmation bias (and other foibles of human judgment) bring us to wage war against one another, time and again.[41] This problem goes back as far as we have written records. As noted in chapter 3, when detailing the run up to the Peloponnesian War between Athens and Sparta that occurred in antiquity, general and historian Thucydides wrote: "For it is a habit of humanity to entrust to careless hope what they long for, and to use sovereign reason to thrust aside what they do not desire."[42]

CHAPTER 7

PATTERNS IN THE STATIC

Nostradamus was a great seer who predicted many major events in the world. Hundreds of years before either of them was born, Nostradamus predicted the rise of both Napoleon and Hitler in a stunning affirmation of his prescient abilities. In the case of Napoleon, he wrote, "PAU, NAY, LORON will be more of fire than of the blood, To swim in praise, the great one to flee to the confluence. He will refuse entry to the Piuses, The depraved ones and the Durance will keep them imprisoned."[1] The name Napoleon leaps out at you from "PAU, NAY, LORON," doesn't it? More of fire than of blood indicates the modern gun powder–based firearms that Napoleon used as part of the new and modern weaponry of the time.

Refusing entry to the Piuses predicts Napoleon's bold willingness to stand up to the Pope. As if this were not amazing enough, regarding the prediction of Hitler's rise, Nostradamus wrote: "From the depths of the West of Europe, A young child will be born of poor people, He who by his tongue will seduce a great troop; His fame will increase towards the realm of the East."[2] Nostradamus goes on to predict that "Beasts ferocious from hunger will swim across rivers: The greater part of the region will be against the Hister, The great one will cause it to be dragged in an iron cage, When the German child will observe nothing."[3] It is simple to see the incredible predictive power of this phrase. Hitler was born of poor people in Europe; his tongue and famous oratory seduced a whole nation and army. He certainly expanded to the East. Iron cages are obviously the tanks that his army used and the phrase specifies Germany in particular. Nostradamus even names who he is talking about, calling him "Hister," only a single letter off from Hitler.

It is hard to understand how someone could predict the future so well without truly having special powers. Surely, this cannot be just lucky guessing. Indeed, it seems that the world has mysterious forces at work that we simply don't grasp. There are links between things that transcend what we understand, but comprise clear evidence of what medieval scholars called "natural magic," a hidden sympathetic connectedness in the world.

To those who pay careful attention, evidence of such connectedness can be found everywhere. Consider, for example, the hidden significance of the number 129:

- Hitler was born 129 years after Napoleon.
- Hitler took power 129 years after Napoleon took power.
- Hitler invaded Russia 129 years after Napoleon did.
- Hitler was defeated 129 years after Napoleon.
- The *Hindenburg* was a Nazi zeppelin that bore the swastika on its tail, and went up in flames, portending the fire that would be unleashed on Europe by the Third Reich (the *Hindenburg*'s call sign was LZ-129).
- William Shakespeare's 129th Sonnet, which is about lust, power, and destruction, ended with the line "that leads men to hell."

Examining the number 129 more deeply, we first note this number has three digits. Notice that the sum of the first two numbers (1 + 2) equals 3. The last number (9) divided by 3 also equals 3. Thus, we find the number 129 has the number 3 embedded throughout. Applying this number 3 to the only two individuals to conquer Europe (i.e., Hitler and Napoleon) gives us the equation $2 \times 3 = 6$. Remember also that we are talking about groups of three, so three repetitions of this number is 666, which is the number of the beast foretold in the new testament. Surely, if the devil has a hand in anything, then it would be in the massive suffering and evil that transpired in the wars waged by these two men, not to mention the Holocaust. To reinforce this from another level, if using base 6 as a number system, then 129 = 333. Again, applying 333 to two dictators produces 666. Strikingly, one number less than 666 at each digit is 555, which was Hitler's membership number in the Nazi Party.[4]

Evidence of prescient forces in the world are not limited to Nostradamus. Indeed, the very word of God contains hidden connections and patterns that portend future events. In this case, consider the monotheistic Abrahamic God, in particular, the basis for Judaism, Christianity, and Islam. In each of these religions, the ancient text of the Old Testament, the Torah (or first five books of Moses), is recognized as a holy book that has come to us, largely unaltered, from its original written form, in ancient Hebrew and on Torah scrolls. These scrolls provide a narrative of this God and the ancient Israelites and serve as the basis for God's law. The Torah also contains a secret code that is hidden in the text in a web of cryptography, which actually predicts the specific happenings of the universe in general and human society in particular.

"The Code" in the Torah was first discovered by a mathematician named Dr. Eliyahu Rips, but it was made more widely known by a journalist named "Michael Drosnin" in his landmark book entitled *The Bible Code*.[5] The way one finds the code is simple in concept. First, one deletes all the spaces in the Torah so it is a single line of text from start to finish—like one really long word (as it is claimed that God gave the Torah to Moses). Then, one chooses a number and identifies the letters that are found at increments of that number. To use the example of Drosnin, consider the sentence—"Rips explained that each code is a case of adding every fourth." Next, consider if the rule is to read every fourth letter. The letters that emerge are as follows:

"Rips explained that each code is a case of adding every fourth."

In in other words: "READ THE CODE."

In actuality, the number of letters skipped is often quite large, and one makes blocks of text that are each the length of the skipped letters. Thus, one creates a "crossword puzzle" like conformation. One can search the text with a series of skip numbers and look for a skip number that results in a person's name or an event being found somewhere in the text. Then one looks for other words in close proximity to the name or event of interest, using the same skip number. By using this approach, the words "Hitler," "Evil Man," "Nazi and Enemy," and "Slaughter" were all found clustered together in the Torah. Likewise, Eichmann was encoded with "the ovens" and "extermination" and "Zyklon B" (Zyklon B was a gas used by Nazi's to execute prisoners in concentrations camps). "In Germany" was encoded with "Nazis" and "Berlin." "In Auschwitz" was encoded near where the original text of the Torah decrees "an end to all flesh." Words can appear horizontally, vertically, or diagonally, and their letters can also be spaced out with other letters in between.

Both the examples of Nostradamus and *The Bible Code* reveal that hidden patterns and prophecies can predict what is going to happen in the future. Using human ability to find meaningful patterns, which now is enhanced by powerful computers, we can fully embrace these approaches, refine and understand them, and increase judicious use of them to predict and control the world. We need to ignore the skeptics who would doubt such clear connections—common sense tells us this could not be a coincidence and could not happen by chance alone. How many future disasters will we sit by and idly allow to occur when the evidence of what is going to happen is right in front of us?

Or maybe not. Maybe we should not fully embrace approaches that notice individual coincidence and then combine these coincidences to discover deeper patterns in the world. Maybe overindulging in such thinking leads to the deranged ramblings of a mad mind, a psychotic obsession with connections and conspiracy, consumed with finding deep and profound meaning in the odd coincidences of chance and acting with definitive effect based upon a simple misinterpretation of random noise. How could such be the case, especially in light of the profound evidence of Nostradamus's and *The Bible Code*'s abilities to predict? This is just the tip of the iceberg regarding prophecy.

Mistaking the Likely for the Seemingly Impossible: Misjudging the Numerator

The more unlikely an event seems, the more it draws our attention when it does occur and the more compelled we feel to explain why it happened. This just makes good sense. If the world is not behaving according to the rules we understand, perhaps we misunderstand the rules. Our attention should be drawn to unlikely occurrences because new knowledge comes from our attempts to understand contradictions.

Sometimes what seems to be impossible is actually highly probable. A famous example of this is found with playing the lottery (i.e., the lottery fallacy).[6] It is well understood that it is incredibly unlikely that any particular person will win the lottery. For example, the chance of any one ticket winning the Powerball lottery (the particular lottery analyzed in this chapter) is 1/292,000,000.[7] This explains why so much attention is paid to the winners. Where did they buy their ticket? Did they see a fortune teller before buying their ticket, or do they have a history of showing psychic abilities? Do they have any special rituals they carry out before buying a ticket? It is a natural tendency to try to explain how such an unlikely event could have occurred. If we can identify a reason, then perhaps understanding it will help us win the lottery, too.

The lottery fallacy is not restricted to good things happening. Explanations also are sought to explain bad things. Some people are struck by lightning more than once, which seems just too unlikely to accept as random chance. There must be some explanation. Inevitably, it is speculated that the person may have some weird mutant trait that makes them attract electricity, or they carry certain metals on their person or have titanium prosthetics in their body. Perhaps they have been cursed by a mystical force or God has forsaken them.

The lottery fallacy can be understood as a form of mistaking one probability for another, or to continue with our theme from part 1, to mistake one fraction for another. One can express the odds of winning the lottery as the fraction (1/292,000,000), in which the numerator is the single number combination that wins and the denominator is all possible number combinations. The fallacy arises because we tend to notice only the one person with the one ticket who won the lottery. This is not the only person playing the lottery, however, and it is not the only ticket. How many tickets are purchased for any given drawing? The exact number changes, because more tickets are sold when the jackpot is higher; however, a typical drawing includes about 300 million tickets sold. Of course, some of the tickets sold must be duplicates, given that only 292 million combinations are possible. Moreover, if every possible combination were being purchased, then someone would win every drawing. In reality, about 50 percent of the drawings have a winner; thus, we can infer that, on average, 146 million different number combinations are purchased.

Of course, the news does not give us a list of all the people who *did not* win. Can you imagine the same headline every week, "299,999,999 People Failed to Win the Lottery, Again!" (names listed online at www.thisweeksloosers.com).[8] No, the news only tells us that there was a winner, and sometimes who the winner was. When we ask ourselves, "What are the odds of that person winning?" we are asking the wrong question and referring to the wrong fraction. The odds of that particular person winning are 1/292,000,000. By chance alone, that person should win the lottery once every 2,807,692 years that they consistently play (assuming two drawings per week). What we should be asking is "What are the odds of *any* person winning?"

In probability, the chances of either one thing or another thing happening are the sum of the individual probabilities. So, assuming no duplicate tickets, if only a single person were playing the lottery, then the odds of having a winner are 1/292,000,000. If two people are playing, the odds of having a winner are 2/292,000,000. If 1,000 people are playing, then the odds are 1,000/292,000,000.[9] Once we consider that 146 million different number combinations are purchased, the top of the fraction (numerator) becomes incredibly large, and the odds that someone will win are quite high. When we marvel at the fact that someone has won the lottery, we mistake the real fraction (146,000,000/292,000,000) for the fraction (1/292,000,000)—that is, we are misjudging the numerator. What seems like an incredibly improbable event is actually quite likely. The human tendency to make this mistake is related to the availability heuristic, as described in chapter 2. Only the winner is "available" to our minds, and not all the many people who did not win.

Similarly, the odds of twice being struck by lightning over the course of one's life are one in nine million. Because 7.9 billion people live on Earth, it is probable that 833 people will be hit by lightning twice in their lives (at least).[10] As with the lottery example, our attention is drawn only to those who are struck by lightning. We fail to consider how many people never get struck. Just as it is unlikely that any one particular person will win the Powerball lottery, it is highly unlikely that no one will win the lottery after a few drawings, just given the number of people playing. Likewise, it is very unlikely that any one person will be twice hit by lightning, but it is even more unlikely that no one will, given the number of people in the world.

So, when we puzzle over such amazing things as someone winning the lottery or being twice struck by lightning, we actually are trying to explain why a highly probable thing happened, which really requires no explanation at all. The rules of the world are working exactly as we understand them, but we are mistaking the highly likely for the virtually impossible.

Finding Patterns in the Static: How Misjudging the Numerator Leads Us to Find Significant Patterns and Associations in Random Noise

Consider the article printed by NBC News on their "Today News" page entitled "Citrus Christ? Cheesus? 13 Religious Sightings: God Is Everywhere—Including an Orange, a Cat's Fur and a Bag of Cheetos."[11] In this article, pictures are shown of actual sightings of Jesus Christ, the Virgin Mary, or Crucifixes in everyday objects. Such sightings happen from time to time, and when they do, they can stir up much interest and excitement. Some of the faithful even make pilgrimages to see the miraculous appearance of the holy images.

In our normal human experience, we encounter a great many things, almost endless things, most of which we do not notice. Certain things stand out, however, and humans have an incredible capacity to recognize particular patterns. This tendency was termed "patternicity" by Michael Shermer in his book *How We Believe*, in which he gives an excellent description of the breadth and depth of these tendencies.[12]

Faces are at the top of the list of things we tend to recognize. This is no mystery. Imagine if we could not recognize when we were looking at a human or an animal that was looking back at us. It would be a serious impediment to our survival.[13] Our ability to find faces in everyday objects, and even assign them emotion, is both impressive and humorous. We are face-finding machines and can identify them in a great many places (see figure 7.1). When your brain recognizes something that is not really there, it is called pareidolia—and humans are quite good at it.

So, the question is whether religious icons actually are present in oranges, cat fur, and Cheetos. Or is human pareidolia just playing tricks on us? This leads us to ask how likely it is for material things to have patterns that can be recognized as religious icons by chance alone. At first consideration, that chance seems pretty low; after all, we all look at things all the time and most of us never see a religious icon. Like the lottery fallacy in which we do not appreciate the number of people who play the lottery but do not win, we also are not mindful

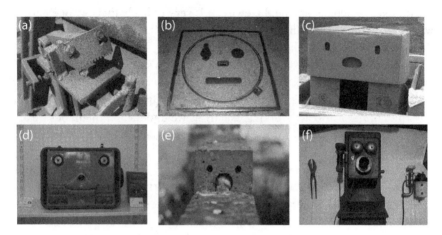

7.1 Six images that cause pareidolia.

Source: Image (e) by Harry Grout. All other photos are in the public domain. Courtesy of Wikimedia Commons.

of the vast number of things we look at and in which we fail to see the image of a religious figure.

How many different images fall on your eyes over the course of an entire year? This would be difficult to calculate, but it cannot be a small number. Now multiply this by 350 million Americans. The additive number of images seen by Americans alone each year must be staggering—not to mention the other 7.5 billion people globally. What are the odds that just a handful of these images would contain a pattern that the human mind might recognize as resembling the Virgin Mary or Christ?

Even if the odds that a pattern that resembled the Virgin Mary would be present in some mundane object were one in a trillion (1/1,000,000,000,000) and 350 million Americans each saw 73,000 visual fields per year (a very small number; just 200 per day), then 26 sightings would be made each year by chance alone based solely on random arrangements of things in the environment. If only a few of those were publicized each year, this would be consistent with the occasional reporting of sightings that occurs.

This is another example of confusing one fraction for another. The fraction we are so impressed by is the probability that in this particular orange, on this particular day, after cutting it at this particular point, we would see an image we recognize as the Virgin Mary. The correct fraction is the probability that, in any of the endless images we see over our lifetimes, we would ever encounter any arrangement of visual stimuli that looked like any one of the religious icons we would recognize. Multiply this number by the millions of people using social media who would post such an image for other people to see. The only thing that actually is highly improbable would be if people *did not* see religious icons—that would require an explanation.

So, can we unequivocally rule out that the One God, the creator of all the universe, chooses to be revealed to humans through grilled cheese sandwiches and oranges? No, we cannot rule this out. Perhaps, as the article suggests, God chooses to be revealed to people precisely by appearing in everyday objects. For a humble God, this may very well be the preferred route. After all, it is said that "God works in mysterious ways." What we can guarantee is that by chance alone, such images would be noticed even in the absence of a divine process. When religious icons are identified, it creates the appearance of a miracle that defies explanation by any means other than the divine. In reality, no explanation is needed because it is all but certain to occur entirely on its own.

In addition to recognizing entities, humans are the consummate finders of associations in nature. Noticing an association between eating a certain berry and getting sick, and then avoiding the berry offers a distinct advantage over failing to notice such a link. Recognizing that planting seeds in the ground results in crops growing gives a huge advantage over failing to recognize this connection. It is easy to see how such traits would give a reproductive advantage and thus be selected by evolution. So, here we are. To maximize the ability to detect patterns and associations, however, one must pay the price of detecting patterns and associations that do not really exist. We are highly effective in noticing associations, and because we observe so many different things in our lives, we also notice associations that occur by random chance.

In his delightfully humorous work, *Spurious Correlations*,[14] author Tyler Vigen shows in expert fashion that if one examines enough things, amazingly strong and ridiculous correlations can be found. For example, Vigen notes a high correlation between the "Age of Miss America" in any given year and "Murder by steam, hot vapors, and hot objects"; a striking correlation (0.992558) between the "divorce rate in Maine" and the "per capita consumption of margarine" in the United States. The list goes on and on, and I recommend you take a look at it. It illustrates what happens if enough data are analyzed. In this case, we notice the hits and discount the misses, which is just another way of misperceiving the fraction. What Vigen did not report was every example of two things that *did not* correlate, which would have been a much larger book. If, however, one takes this into account, then the spurious correlations are the inevitable result of having examined enough things.[15]

The algorithm that discovered *The Bible Code*, described at the beginning of this chapter, revealed the same result as Tyler Vigen's humorous exercise. The number of combinations of letters that resulted in gibberish was so immense that the emergence of some words of meaning was inevitable by chance alone.[16] Moreover, more than a few years have passed since the Torah was written and a great many events have transpired, which profoundly increases the odds that word combinations could apply to some world event. Statistician Brendan McKay and colleagues demonstrated this fact to great effect by applying *The Bible Code* algorithm to the text of *Moby-Dick*, which clearly foretold the assassinations of Abraham Lincoln, Indira Gandhi, John F. Kennedy, Dr. Martin Luther King, Jr., and Yitzhak Rabin.[17]

Some people responded to the results of the *Moby-Dick* exercise not with a recognition of the error that had been made in *The Bible Code*, but rather, by concluding that the Bible represents just one of many texts that includes important messages. Perhaps a concerted effort to search all published literature using such methods, and then changing our entire life strategy based on these predictions, would be the best approach—or maybe not. The response to the *Moby-Dick* exercise reveals how deeply seated our tendency to believe in these patterns actually is.

This same issue of mistaking a very large fraction for a small one is why Nostradamus appears prescient and why the number 129 seems to have mystical importance. It is simply an issue of being creative enough to find coincidences and connections, without being aware of the vast number of things that do not correlate and we do not notice. This is not unlike Tyler Vigan's spurious correlations. A lot of events have transpired since Nostradamus made his predictions, and more are happening every day. His predictions are so vague, abstract, and numerous that they can be twisted to fit a great many circumstances. The numerator is expanded even more with the help of the human imagination and flexibility of language. The list of all the things that could be predicted from Nostradamus's writing that *have not* occurred is essentially endless. In other words, it is extremely likely, almost inevitable, that many of Nostradamus's predictions will appear to have come true, even if he had absolutely no prescient abilities.

Summary

When an event occurs, the more improbable it was to happen, the more reason we have to look for some explanation. If we can find a cause, then the happening is no longer unlikely and our understanding of the event may be useful. The accurate predictions of world events that *The Bible Code* reveals are not unlikely if an all-knowing God created them for us to find. In that case, *The Bible Code* truly could help us in the future. The success of Nostradamus's predictions is not unlikely if he actually was clairvoyant, and his quatrains could be a great guide. Consider that it is far more likely for someone to be struck twice by lightening if they live on a property that attracts electricity. In that case, we would be well advised to avoid that property. A specific person winning the lottery is more likely if their good luck ritual actually works, and thus we might want to try this ritual ourselves. The strategy of finding a cause that explains why otherwise unlikely events occur, however, presupposes that they actually are unlikely.

The issue explored in this chapter is not the fact that we notice things, but rather the likelihood of occurrence that we assign to the things we notice. In other words, a one in a million outcome is pretty unlikely if you only try something once; however, that same outcome is highly likely if you try something a million times. We are prone to confuse the latter for the former by focusing on instances in which an event does occur and by ignoring all the times it does not. We invent explanations for why a highly likely thing actually happened, which leads us to believe both in phenomena that do not exist and to identify causes that are not real. In these cases, the explanation for why an extremely unlikely thing happened is simply because it actually was not unlikely. That is all. Sometimes hidden causes *can* be found for otherwise unlikely things, and it is beneficial to seek out those causes.

Humans are just bad at telling the difference.

CHAPTER 8

ALTERNATIVE AND NEW AGE BELIEFS

A great many individuals and systems of belief claim the ability to tap into special powers. Powers may come from knowledge of nature (e.g., astrology), use of particular mystical items (e.g., tarot cards, runes, or crystals), or an inborn gift (e.g., clairvoyance). It is easy to find people to read your aura or your chakra, predict your future, speak with the dead, or claim to have other astounding abilities.

People are fairly intelligent and grounded in reality, in general. Some personality types accept fantastic claims easier than others. Still, given how astounding many claims are, most people would not accept them without some pretty impressive evidence. This is why practitioners often start interactions with a demonstration of their abilities. Psychics, for example, often start off showing that they know specific things about a person they have never met; things they could not possibly know by ordinary means.[1] It is uncanny, unbelievable really, all of the details that they can provide about the person being "read". It is so astounding, in fact, that psychic abilities seem indisputably demonstrated. Even with some skepticism, people who witness these powers are left with no other viable explanation—in fact, no other explanation at all—other than authentic clairvoyance. There is just no other way the psychic could know what they know.

Many skeptics dismiss psychics' claims out of hand. However, such skepticism may seem unfounded and closed minded to those who have experienced the meaningful process of being read. If a person has never met you or anyone you know and is able to "read" you such that they have knowledge that they could not reasonably guess by chance, then this provides proof of their clairvoyance—especially if they can do it over and over again.

The evidence seems straightforward. The fact that the person being read experiences the power of the psychic is not in question. What is in question is whether this experience proves, or is even any evidence at all, of underlying psychic powers. The conclusion of clairvoyant powers assumes that the psychic could not have reasonably guessed by chance alone. At first consideration, such chance guessing seems so improbable as to be impossible. But what if people misunderstood the probability of guessing correctly?

A Real-Life Mentalist at Work

A psychic stands before a crowd of 300 people at a public demonstration of mind reading. Let's set aside situations where the psychic has secretly obtained knowledge of the subjects.[2] Let's also guarantee that no one in the audience is a "confederate"—that is, a partner of the psychic who fakes being read. We stipulate that the psychic has never met anyone in the audience and really knows nothing specific about them. The psychic looks up at the audience, holding his head in his hands with intense concentration and says:

> I'm picking up a strange image. I'm not sure, but I'm going to go ahead with what I'm seeing . . . I'm seeing a clown, yes. A man dressed as a clown. He's standing in a graveyard and he's putting flowers on the graves. Does that mean anything to anyone? . . . and I see the name Stanley."

Amazingly, a woman stands up, looking terrified, and screams out:

> There's no way you could have known that! There was an old man in my home-town who used to dress-up in a clown costume and put flowers on the graves in the town cemetery. My name is Cindy but for some reason that guy always called me Stanley! How the hell did you know that?

This story is incredible and is exactly the type of experience that would convince many people who witnessed it of the clear existence of psychic pow-ers. It may even convince people who just heard it. Indeed, this story really happened in a demonstration by a renowned mentalist at a convention hall in Atlanta in 2012.

There is one major problem with using this as an example of psychic ability. The clairvoyant in this case is Mark Edward and he is *not* a psychic; rather, he is a professional magician who fools people for a living. Moreover, he performed this act as part of a lecture to specifically explain why highly accurate readings by psychics are not conclusive evidence of psychic abilities—and they may provide no evidence at all.[3]

If Edward actually has no special powers, then how did he accomplish the amazing reading of the clown in the graveyard? He couldn't have done this by just chance alone—or could he? Edward's explanation reveals that he did this precisely by chance alone, and that the seeming improbability of the event is an error of misjudging likelihood. Remember, he did not point specifically at one particular woman and say—I see a clown in a graveyard in your past. Rather, he made the statement to the whole audience, such that if anyone in the room had a history of a clown in a graveyard, then they would have raised their hand.

Admittedly, a clown in a graveyard is a pretty obscure example. Edwards points out that a psychic would more commonly say something like this: "I'm seeing someone's husband. Did someone's husband pass to the other side from lung cancer here tonight? After which any psychic worth his or her salt would expect to see dozens of up-raised tear-filled eyes."

When someone in the audience pops up and confirms the psychic's prediction is correct, it seems amazing because it seems so unlikely, and it seems so unlikely because people focus on the odds of the psychic knowing such a thing about that particular person. One is mistaking the fraction that is relevant to the situation. The real fraction is the aggregate probability, which is found by adding up all the individual probabilities—in other words all the people in the room. This results in massively expanding the numerator of the probability fraction and converting an improbable event into a likely one.

If the odds of a person having a particular event in their life are 1/300, and 300 people are in the audience, then when the psychic asks, "has this event happened to anyone?" it is not surprising that someone says yes. The probability is not whether one person had a father die from cancer, it is whether *anyone* had a father die from cancer. The probability fraction is not 1/300, it is 300/300, which is 100 percent.

The psychic sprays predictions across the entire crowd, and then the person (or people) to whom they apply identify themselves to the psychic. The audience focuses on the person (or people) the predictions work for and ignores everyone else (i.e., the entire rest of the crowd). This is exactly the same issue as was explored in the previous chapter with lotteries, lightning strikes, *The Bible Code*, and Nostradamus. In this case, however, it is not just the person doing it on their own, it is a partnership between the New Age practitioner and all of the subjects.

How can we explain the clown in the graveyard, and even the name Stanley? This is not lung cancer; this is weird, obscure, and quite specific. Doesn't this example bring us back to a very low probability? It certainly is less likely than guessing at something common like lung cancer, or simply having lost a father. That said, the life experience of 300 people is a massive dataset. Moreover, the likelihood of a psychic "hit" goes up dramatically because people will twist and abstract their experiences to make them fit. As Edwards goes on to explain, unlike magicians where everyone wants him or her to fail so they can uncover the secret of the trick, with fortune tellers, people tend to want them to succeed.[4] They want it to be real. He explains:

> As in psychic readings, they *want* the performer to succeed and in most cases will do anything they can to help out. People *need* to believe. They may not necessarily need to believe a rabbit comes out of a hat, but when it comes to death and the hereafter, an audience of believers will consistently make connections of the most bizarre and ridiculous kind.

This means that people will work with the psychic to give a liberal interpretation to what constitutes a correct prediction. They might say something like "My uncle loved the movie *Tombstone*, so he had a link to graveyards and he was a joker and we always called him the family clown, so yes! He was a clown in a graveyard." This is a further example of modifying the fraction. By expanding what can be counted as "a hit," we dramatically increase the odds of making a correct guess.

The question is no longer "How likely is it that the psychic could have guessed that fact about me?" Now the question is "How likely is it that the psychic could say something that I could twist and contort my life experience to fit through metaphor and abstraction?" It is the opposite of the no-true-Scotsman fallacy in which anything that does not confirm the rule is excluded. In this case, the numerator of the fraction (things that count as hits) is expanded to include a great many things that have no business being there.

But with the clown in the graveyard, the woman did not need to twist things at all. She really did grow up around a guy who literally dressed as a clown, went to graveyards, and called her Stanley. Even Mark Edward admits he was surprised by this hit, but he also noted that he always throws some odd predictions out to the crowd (although usually he does not get a response). According to his explanation of how taking an occasional risk can only help a psychic, if you use enough high-probability statements (e.g., I sense someone who has lost a father), typically there will be many hits. In addition, more hits will be guaranteed by making statements that essentially cannot be false. For example, in reading someone's personality the psychic may say, "You are usually a very reasonable person, but at times, when under stress, you can become grumpy." To whom of us would that not apply?[5] Setting aside what others may think, how many people do not think they are reasonable? And how many of us have never been grumpy when stressed?

In this background of hits, having an occasional miss can increase credibility, because a perfect hit rate would seem more suspicious and might lead people to thinking it was a trick. Again, as explained by Edward referring to the clown in the graveyard:

> It's always good business to throw in two or three ridiculous bits like this. When a psychic is wrong, it makes it more believable. The audience reasons (wrongly) that if what they have heard was a trick, then like a magician, the performer would have been dead-on right. But since they were wrong and got no response, it must be something real. Why else would he or she say that?[6]

Importantly, the real probability of Edward's correct prediction of the clown in the graveyard is not just the chance of 300 people happening to have a clown in a graveyard somewhere in their past. Edward is telling us only of the one time that a crazy guess he threw out to the crowd was a hit. The real number of people being asked includes all the times that Edward threw out a crazy idea and he did not have a hit at all (e.g., most of the time). In this case, the real numerator is all of the life experiences of all the people encountered over the entire career of a professional stage mentalist. That is the real fraction to consider, and the probability it describes is pretty likely.

We also must consider that people typically have poor intuition about how likely it is that things are going to happen, in general. Consider if a psychic entered a room of 30 people, looked about the room, and said, "I am feeling a synchronicity of spirit here, a fundamental link between two people—yes, I can see it. Two people in this room have the identical birthday, and it joins their energy." The psychic then has each person in the room state their birthday, and sure enough, two people were born on the very same day.[7]

This is one of my favorite examples of poor estimation of probability. Consider birthdays. If we include February 29 (to account for leap years), then we have 366 possible birthdays. So, to be 100 percent sure that at least two people in a room have an identical birthday, we need to have at least 367 people in the room. So how many people would have to be in the room for there to be a 50 percent chance of two people sharing the same birthday?

The answer is not half of 367 (or 184).[8] The correct answer is only 23 people. To be clear, we are not saying that with 23 people, if you called out a specific birthday, then there is a 50 percent chance that two people were born on that day. It would take 253 people to accomplish that probability. Rather, we are saying that for 23 people, there is a 50 percent chance that two of them will have been born on the same day, where all days are possible.[9] In many cases, when people see what are believed to be amazing coincidences, the coincidences actually are not that unlikely.

So what happens when you visit a psychic one on one, and not in a crowd? How might we misunderstand probability in that setting? The entire life experiences of 300 people are now lacking; it's just you. The psychic may say something like, "I am sensing a person from your past with a first letter of their name being a J? or an M? or an S? or maybe a D? " Amazingly, your father's name is David. You forget the missed J, M, and S and focus on the D. Still, only four guesses (out of 26 letters)—that is pretty fantastic. Well, when you add up names and frequencies, it turns out that 40 percent of names begin with one of these four letters.[10] Now consider how many people are in your past. Even if we limit this number to people of high significance (i.e., family and loves ones), it is likely no fewer than 11 (four grandparents, two parents, siblings, close friends, boyfriends/ girlfriends). The odds of any one of them not having a name that begins with such a letter is 6/10 (0.6) = 60 percent. The odds of none of them having a name that begins with such a letter is 0.6^{11} = 0.0036. In other words, a psychic will fail to get a hit in only 1 out of every 276 times the psychic uses this approach—and that is assuming that clients have only 11 people in their past, or in other words over their entire lives. If a person has 40 people in their past (a very reasonable number), then the psychic is more likely to win the Powerball lottery after playing a single time than to *not* get a hit in response to this question.[11]

More than 50 percent of deaths of the elderly are due to heart disease or cancer of some kind. Close to 100 percent of people who have lost a parent have at least some regret over something regarding the parent's death. Let's say a psychic is talking to a 70-year-old client; the probability is very high that both parents are dead. So, if a psychic said, "I am hearing the spirit of a dead parent (client nods yes), a mother or father (client also nods yes), who died from heart disease or maybe cancer (client usually nods yes). I am sensing some deep regret in you surrounding their passing (client nods yes). The psychic has now established their powers and has the client working with them. Off to the races they go with the full force of both questions geared to increase the likelihood of "a hit" and confirmation bias to grease the rails.

In addition to the psychic asking questions likely to get a positive result, subjects work hard with the psychic, unbeknownst to them, to increase the likelihood of the correct guesses. This is what Edward was referring to when he said "people will do anything they can to help out." This is an entirely unconscious process and people do not know they are doing it, despite the fact they are extremely good at it.

Even if the psychic guesses wrong, the client will exert great effort to make it right.

"I'm sensing a mother or father who died from heart disease," the physic says.

"Oh, who you are sensing is my uncle Bill, " explains the client. "He was my uncle, but he was always *like* a father to me, and he died from pneumonia but really once his wife had died he just lost the will to live, so he died from a broken heart, which is basically heart disease. It is definitely my uncle Bill who you are sensing."

The client's father did not die of heart disease, but somehow, an uncle who died from pneumonia became a father who died of heart disease. By using abstraction and imagination, experience can be adapted to almost any prediction. Humans are creative beings. In terms of a fraction, this is another case of reclassifying a great many things so that they qualify to be included in the numerator. One is increasing the probability to essentially 100 percent.

It is also somewhat ironic that most psychics pose their predictions in the form of questions, and not statements. This is because they are seeking hits, upon which they then follow up with additional questions, and they can back off of any misses. This process also creates a rhythm by which the client is cooperating and working with the psychic to find the hits. With that understanding, we return to an insightful statement from Edward.

> If psychics were real, they wouldn't need to ask even a single question. They would just know. Period. End of story. Yet if we listen to any of the latest crop of psychic mediums in a live situation and not in edited television formats, that's all they do. Its non-stop question after question after question.[12]

The evidence of psychic abilities usually comes from reading a person's past. In contrast, psychics seldom make specific predictions about the future. When they do, they are usually wrong. Through an abstract twisting of events, it may look like they got something right, just like the father who died of heart disease becoming an uncle who died of pneumonia.

Correct predictions also can be manufactured by "moving the goal posts," which is a way of changing the rules for what counts as a correct prediction, so that "a hit" is inevitable. Someone may predict an earthquake will occur in the next three years—an earthquake does occur (but five years later)—even so, this is counted as a hit. Or a cyclone hits Bali, and the psychic claims that this is what they were really sensing, but the harmonics of the universe where slightly distorted, so the cyclone appeared to them as an earthquake. Moving the goal posts essentially allows predictions to be "I predict that something will happen at some point," which is a certainty.

Science, Skepticism, and New Age Beliefs

The label New Age encompasses a great many things, and it is impossible to precisely define it in a way that includes all belief constructs.[13] In typical usage, however, New Age may refer to areas, such as spiritualism (including the channeling of spirits), astrology, clairvoyance, psychics, tarot cards, the power of runes, the power of crystals, and a great many other practices and beliefs of a similar theme. Whereas the New Age movement specifically refers to developments in beliefs since the 1970s, many of these beliefs originate from ancient systems from multiple cultures and pertain to both natural and supernatural effects. Such beliefs have been with us as long as we have had records and likely as long as humans have walked the Earth.

Scientific and New Age approaches often are framed as polar opposites, with New Age approaches being labeled as "pseudoscience" by scientists and skeptics. Although many distinctions have been argued as to what defines science and demarcates it from other approaches to knowledge, science most often is distinguished by its emphasis on data. Data, however, are just a form of experience. New Age approaches are no less based on observation and evidence than is science.[14] Indeed, most New Age approaches place a premium on experience. Scientific and New Age approaches, however, differ in the types of experience that they value, or even allow.[15]

Practitioners of New Age systems tend to accept personal experience, in and of itself, as the gold standard of evidence. In contrast, scientists are trained to doubt their own experience (and that of others) and to question whether what their senses are telling them is "real." Scientists also question whether their instruments are correctly measuring nature or whether the instruments are distorting or even generating a measurement. Scientists are trained to question and doubt if their interpretation of experience is correct. This is not radical skepticism. Scientists do not doubt everything no matter what the evidence shows; rather, they doubt judiciously and actively test their doubts by experimental means that have the ability to further support or refute their beliefs.

Skeptical questioning of experience is not generally found in New Age approaches, and in most cases, is anathema to their practices, as will be expanded on next. This is not to imply that New Age practitioners accept all things without question. Clearly, such is not the case, and they are likely to reject many more belief systems than they accept, including other New Age beliefs. I am referring specifically to doubting personal experience as an entity. Unlike science, New Age systems generally lack suspicion and skepticism about experience itself. New Age practices do not typically have what Lee McIntyre has called "the scientific attitude."[16]

To be clear, scientists and skeptics do not question that powerful experiences are had as a result of New Age practices. Clearly, people experience the effects of auras, chakras, crystals, and universal harmonics, as well as the predictive power of psychics. Rather, the question is whether the experience was caused by actual "real" things (called chakras) or whether the experience was just a process internal to our minds that allowed us to perceive chakras, without the existence of a "real" chakra. The experience of chakras is undeniably real. But are actual chakras causing the experience, or is it just an experience?

Each of us has had dreams. The dream was "real" in the sense that we had the dream, which is to say we experienced it. However, most people recognize that the dream did not actually occur outside of us dreaming it. In other words, we distinguish between experiences that are the result of happenings external to ourselves from the experiences that originate within our own minds. Even for those who believe in "the power of dreams" to predict what may happen in the "real world," it is still recognized that the dream is not the same as direct experience of an external reality, as we would have when awake.

We do not need to have a dream to generate experience from within our own minds. A good hypnotist, working with a willing client, can get the client to experience a wide variety of amazing physical sensations through simple suggestion. So, the mind is quite capable of actively generating experiences on its own not linked to an external cause. We also do this to ourselves all the time without any external suggestion. If you are camping in the woods, and you get it into your head that ants may be in your sleeping bag, even if there are no ants, good luck not interpreting every little itch as a bug crawling over your body.

Of course, humans can (and do) test their experience with external validations. If you feel an ant crawling up your leg, you investigate. If you don't find an ant, after investigating several "false alarms," you may conclude that you are just imagining things and then ignore itches going forward. Our observations of the external world work as metrics for the validity of how we interpret experience; this is the normal everyday human version of scientific research. However, this leads us back to the main theme of this book: In what circumstances do humans misperceive the external world, such that they "mistake" incorrect interpretations of experience as "proof" of their beliefs.

What about the effects of crystals, for example? People may believe in the power of crystals to heal because they have experienced the medical benefit themselves and have witnessed the effects they have on others. They may even "feel" the power of the crystals when they are placed on their skin. The question, however, is whether the crystal really is doing something to us or whether we are doing something to ourselves. Is the "feeling" of energy coming from the crystal just a form of self-hypnosis, much like the "feeling" of ants climbing up your leg when no ants are there? In this case, checking whether the ant is really there comes in the form of seeing whether people really get better when they have crystal therapy. Although most people can tell whether or not an ant is really crawling on them, because of the types of problems detailed in part 1 and in this chapter, it is difficult to tell whether crystals are working just by passive observation. Scientific approaches are specifically designed to test questions such as these and to compensate for human tendencies to misperceive.

Science makes use of controlled trials under particular conditions. If you truly believe that a certain kind of crystal gives health, then to test this theory, one must find a large group of sick people and give half of them crystal therapy and withhold crystal therapy from the other half. The patients need to be randomly assigned to the two groups such that no difference exists between the groups other than whether or not they are getting the therapy. The patients not getting crystal therapy need to believe they are being given the same treatment using "fake crystals," so that none of the patients know whether they are getting the real therapy or the placebo therapy. Ideally, those giving the therapy also will not know who is getting real crystals versus fake crystals. If crystal therapy really works, then those treated with the real crystals should have a better outcome than those treated with fake crystals and the difference should be statistically significant (see chapter 10).

Some claims of New Age approaches certainly have held up to this kind of scrutiny. If rigorously tested in this way, and if the results can be repeated by others, then scientists will accept that the effect is real. They may disagree with the theory behind how it happens, but they will acknowledge that it does happen and become enthusiastic to study it further.[17] For the vast majority of New Age claims that have been tested in this way, however, no differences have been found between the groups. In this case, the scientist would reject the claim of the New Age approach. Scientists would not deny that the New Age practitioners experienced the effects they claim. Scientists would only deny that the experience is linked to anything "real" (other than a placebo effect, which is internal to the mind).

New Age practitioners do not typically make empty claims. They are usually supported by evidence, such as a demonstration of clairvoyant mind reading, a long list of sick people who got better after undergoing a certain therapy or engaging in a certain practice or meditation, someone finding love or wealth, or someone finding happiness only after fully embracing a New Age practice. This is evidence, real evidence, and a great deal of it; testimonials of the amazing effects of New Age practices are abundant. To scientists, however, this kind of evidence is incredibly weak, precisely because it is so vulnerable to the types of effects we have been discussing (i.e., chance effects combined with misunderstanding probability and reinforced by confirmation bias). New Age practitioners often accept testimonials of personal experiences as proof whereas scientists require additional investigation specifically designed to control for the types of errors we have been discussing.

The Effects of Testing and Scrutiny

Let us look at this from the New Age point of view. Patients who come to a New Age crystal clinic feel better after treatment. When a controlled trial is run, however, those getting the fake crystals receive the same benefit as those getting the authentic crystals. A clairvoyant can read clients with uncanny accuracy. However, under controlled conditions in which the clairvoyant cannot pick up on any social cues and does not have the feedback to allow for mining of hits and ignoring of misses, the clairvoyant's ability disappears. The New Age practitioners experience their craft working when they do it the way they are accustomed to, but the effect disappears under scientific scrutiny—the magic doesn't happen anymore.

A scientist would conclude that the whole thing was a mistaken interpretation of experience. The effects never existed other than in the imagination of the practitioners. That said, it would be no less logical for the New Age practitioner to conclude that the effect is real but was inhibited by something in the process of testing it. Perhaps the scrutiny of the scientists, the "negative energy" of their skepticism, or simply the conditions of the test prevented the approach from working. Indeed, this is often the response from adherents of a system in the light of scientific studies that do not support their claims. This is where the trouble begins. To the scientist, such a response is simply a slimy dodge, an unwillingness to be rational and to admit that the approach is nonsense. To the New Age practitioner, they have been forced into conditions in which the magic may not work, so they will just avoid that condition and go to where the magic *does* work.

Scientists often dismiss such maneuvers as irrational; however, such need not be the case from a strictly logical point of view. Consider if I was a "magnetist." I held the tenet that magnets are a vehicle of truth, and any studies done in the absence of magnets were susceptible to error and basically worthless. Now consider that I am talking to a scientist who claims that a compass can identify the direction of the North Pole of the Earth—this is an amazing claim. I find this claim to be questionable, however; how can a small needle balanced within a disk actually find North by detecting some invisible force that permeates the Earth? To test this claim in the most rigorous and truthful way, I ask the scientist to demonstrate the compass in the presence of a strong magnet that I bring with me to impart truth on the experiment. Sadly, the compass does not point to the North Pole under my rigorous conditions; it only points at my truth magnet.

I inform the scientist that the claim about compasses was an observational error, and it just does not hold up to my truth condition. The scientist looks at me blankly and then says, "but your magnet prevents the compass from working, it will only point to the North Pole in the absence of a strong magnet." I chuckle knowingly at the scientist's ignorance and naiveté and attempt to explain why no truth can be known outside of the presence of a strong magnet, which is a necessary component of all true knowledge.

To say that the compass works only outside the presence of a magnet is to say that it works only in the absence of rigorous truthful testing. The scientist maintains the claim about compasses and explains that my view is stupid and silly—my approach destroys the effect. I dismiss the scientist's approach and claims as the sad and irrational bumbling of an ignorant person who just does not get how things work or know how to properly analyze the world. Indeed, each of us thinks the other is an idiot.

Skeptics and scientists will say to New Age practitioners, "we tested your approach using specific methods that are required to find correct answers—and using these methods, your claims fail." To the New Age practitioner, the scientist has insisted on holding a strong magnet next to a compass. Of course, an important difference from the magnet analogy is a tremendous amount of strong evidence showing that proper scientific approaches do actually get rid of common human errors, such as those we have been discussing. To a New Age practitioner, however, such evidence may not carry any weight—scientific methods are just a magnet. This is a disagreement over the quality of different kinds of evidence; the scientist values controlled studies and the New Age practitioner favors uncontrolled individual experience.

If one accepts, as the New Age practitioner may claim, that skepticism and scientific evaluation destroys the effect of a New Age approach, this prohibits scientific analysis. Scientists typically do not accept this view, and they hold that the New Age claims are simply false if the effect disappears under scrutiny. Logically, however, evoking the idea that scientific methodologies destroy the effect removes the relevance of scientific data as to whether the New Age claims are false or true. It simply makes them the sort of thing that scientists cannot study.

One strategy that scientists and skeptics employ is to show that they can produce identical effects but by ordinary means without the trappings or process of the New Age belief. In other words, with no "magic." It is not a coincidence that many "debunkers" are professional magicians—that is, individuals trained (for amusement purposes only) to exploit the cognitive and perceptual errors of people to trick them. These debunkers can provide exactly the same experiences (e.g., clairvoyance, spoon bending, telekinesis) by trickery and in the absence of any mystical power. This invalidates the claim that "I know a New Age power exists because I have *experienced* it working." The very same experience can be generated by simple trickery.

When faced with this argument, New Age practitioners often respond that it is a logical fallacy to conclude that New Age practitioners are not truly using New Age powers to accomplish their claims, just because similar outcomes can be mimicked by professional magicians. From a logical point of view, this argument by New Age practitioners is entirely correct, and it must be respected as such. Indeed, one could use cinematographic trickery to make a movie in which it appears that I can perform a perfect quadruple Lutz on ice skates. One could also watch a film of Brandon Mroz actually performing this amazing move, as the first skater to do a quadruple Lutz in an international competition in 2011.[18] Both Mroz and I have generated a film of ourselves doing a quadruple Lutz, but we have done so using very different methods (e.g., he did it with his athletic ability, and I did it with computer-generated graphics technology).

That I have the ability to reproduce his film by other means in no way indicates that he did not really do a quadruple Lutz. As such, the ability of debunkers to produce the same effects as New Age practitioners is equally consistent with the New Age approach being a misinterpretation of experience (as skeptics claim) as it is with the New Age approach being real but achievable by other means as well (as New Age practitioners claim).

Another cultural distinction between science and New Age beliefs is that private evidence typically is given little weight in science. If a scientist cannot describe precise conditions such that the same result can be replicated by someone else, then at the very least, it cannot be studied, and it is likely not a correct observation at all. In many New Age approaches, however, observation is the personal experience that a practitioner had. Consensus is not needed on what was felt by different people; they all felt what they were supposed to feel. It is good and appropriate that everyone's experience should be different because each person is different.

In addition to challenging each other's observations (e.g., reproducing each other's experiments), scientist also directly challenge each other's interpretations. Even if some scientists are not as self-critical as they could be, they directly criticize and challenge other scientists. This occurs in the published literature, in dialog between scientists, at lab meetings and seminars, and at conferences. Such criticism can be animated, vociferous, and even aggressive. This is a significant difference between science and New Age thinking, and it is based on norms that are deeply baked into the respective cultures.

It is a scientific norm to question the interpretation of experience that others put forth. To an outside viewer, this can often seem like a personal attack, but it is not.[19] Rather, it is an attack on the interpretations of experience, and it is an expected and compulsory part of scientific culture. Scientists are not attacking ideas to be mean or just thump their chests; it is part of a reasoned debate with all of the benefits of an interactionist system (as described in chapter 11). In New Age thinking, however, the opposite is true. In this way, we are looking at opposite approaches in which a required virtue in one area is a forbidden breach of etiquette in the other. This point was made with great eloquence by author Karla McLaren, one of the few ambassadors between spiritual and skeptical thought—a rare individual who has lived fully in both worlds. Previously widely respected in New Age culture with multiple publications and an active practice, McLaren was a self-described "card-carrying, aura-wearing, chakra-toting leader of the New Age." In her excellent essay, "Bridging the Chasm Between Two Cultures," referring to New Age culture, she writes:

> Personal attacks are considered an example of emotional imbalance (where your emotions control you), while deep skepticism is considered a form of mental imbalance (where your intellect controls you). Both behaviors are serious cultural no-nos, because both the emotions and the intellect are considered

troublesome areas of the psyche that do very little but keep one away from the (supposedly) true and meaningful realm of spirit.[20]

It is the point of this book that humans tend to misinterpret the world because of problems in understanding properties that take the form of a fraction (such as probabilities, rates, and frequencies). The word "misinterpret" presupposes that a correct interpretation of how the world really is, external to the observer, is the goal. If, however, the goal of New Age practitioners is to have a particular experience that is meaningful to them, then applying some experimental method that invalidates or destroys the experience is the opposite of what the New Age practitioner is trying to accomplish. Skeptics are actively trying to deprive the practitioner of something he or she very much wants, and may sincerely need—that is, the spiritual experience of something larger than themselves and the feelings of connectivity to the universe. It does not matter to the New Age practitioner whether the effects of crystals are "real" from a scientist's point of view. All that matters is that what the practitioner *feels* is real, which is to say what they experience. The New Age attitude might be "just leave me alone to enjoy my experience and stop trying to spoil it!"

It is easy for skeptics to hold the view that all people who sell or promote New Age systems are charlatans and con artists, victimizing the consumers of their system. As discussed in the next section, that need not be the case, and such scenarios are not what this book is primarily about. This book is about the genuine beliefs of people and how innumeracy and misunderstanding of probability contributes to such beliefs. However, the sociopathic victimization of vulnerable people does require comment.

Even for those who peddle New Age systems they know to be nonsense, one might ask, what harm is there really? If the customer wants or needs the experience, and the New Age system gives them the real experience they seek, what is the problem? Are you also going to attack people who run movie theaters, or who sell virtual reality gear and games that also are providing an experience that isn't "real"? Well, a few big differences are worth noting.

Regrettably, when New Age practitioners sell experience, they often are also selling the belief that it actually is real. That this may be what the consumer is looking for does not mitigate the harm that can be done. Such beliefs can motivate all manner of behavior and decision making that alter lives, and it can come at a high cost. In some cases, New Age consumers are profoundly victimized, giving over their life savings and even their personal freedom. Those who swallow the tenets of a New Age system involving medical therapy for terminal illness not only pay in terms of their money but also pay in terms of their lives, to a seller who knows all too well that the claims are nonsense and that they are purposefully fooling the victim. This is a different and disgusting practice that is morally deplorable as well as criminal. The psychology behind why people are so susceptible to con artists is outside the scope of this book; however, the errors in human perception described in this book are likely a substantial part of the equation.

A Clash of Cultures: A Clash of Views

Both scientists and New Age practitioners may each view their role as simultaneously helping people themselves and protecting people from victimization by others. How could both sides have the same intentions and goals but be acting in such stark opposition? This answer comes down to a clash of views that emerges from a class of cultures and norms of belief and evidence. Let's take accepted medical therapies versus New Age therapies for disease, as an example.

Scientists and skeptics who doubt New Age claims are genuinely trying to prevent victimization of people who, in their view, are being duped by charlatans, while missing mainstream medical therapies that really work.[21] Conversely, New Age practitioners may view the scientists and skeptics as trying to victimize people who are being duped into spending large sums of money on mainstream therapies by a conspiracy of the juggernaut of corporate big pharma and establishment institutions, while missing New Age therapies that really work. How often have you seen an internet ad for the "cure that doctors don't want you to know about"? Just as scientists and skeptics accuse New Age beliefs of substituting a fake therapy for one that works, New Age believers may make the same charge against mainstream scientists.

When the scientists and skeptics who test New Age beliefs challenge the claims being made, they typically view the practitioners as culpable and the consumers as victims. It is often assumed that if consumers are being fooled by practitioners, then the practitioners must have set out to perpetrate a fraud. This view can only be reinforced by famous instances in which this has clearly occurred.[22] However, this need not be the case, and in many instances it is likely that the practitioners truly believe in the effects of what they are practicing.

Professional practitioners of New Age beliefs are no less susceptible to misperceiving the fraction than are the consumers. In this case, the practitioners are focusing on the hits and ignoring the misses they achieve with their clients—expanding the numerator of the probability fraction and increasing their perception of the likelihood of correct predictions or favorable outcomes. Remember, it is a partnership, with two-way communication. New Age practitioners can be entirely rational and base their opinions on evidence in the form of experience. They have clear evidence that what they are doing is really working; they have the reports and testimonials of those they are helping. Returning to McLaren's insights, she writes:

I started out in my youth, knowing (through direct experience) that the things I learned in the New Age and metaphysics were true, and that naysayers were just that . . . My empirical experience "proved" the validity of things like psychic skills, auras, chakras, contact with the dead, astrology, and the like—I had very little in my intellectual arsenal at the time to help me understand what was truly occurring.

She continues:

I didn't understand that I had long used a form of cold reading in my own work! I was never taught cold reading and I never intended to defraud any-one—I simply picked up the technique through cultural osmosis . . . I was never in the field to scam anyone—and neither were any of my friends or col-leagues. I worked in the field because I have a deep and abiding concern for people, and an honest wish to be helpful in my own culture.[23]

It is essential to make a distinction between claims around experience and claims around objective effects. Many New Age claims go far beyond subjec-tive experience. For example, if a claim is made that a New Age therapy cures cancer, this is not simply an issue of experience or perspective. The cancer will or will not be cured, the patient will or will not die from the disease, and death is not simply a state of mind. It is in this context that the types of errors we are discussing are most dangerous. These errors literally cost people their lives.

Based upon how they are carried out and the culture in which they find themselves, New Age claims are particularly susceptible to the types of errors we have been discussing. By prioritizing private experience over controlled scientific methods meant to mitigate error, the practices inevitably fall prey to the prevailing human tendency to be fooled. Indeed, New Age practices and culture guarantee that errors in perception will continue in perpetuity, because mechanisms for them to be tested and rejected are limited.

This does not mean that all New Age beliefs are necessarily untrue. From a logical point of view, one cannot make that claim. It is correct to conclude, however, that because of the types of errors we have been discussing, it is guar-anteed that many New Age beliefs will exist that truly appear to work, when in reality they have no merit whatsoever. At the end of the day, what are we to do and what are we to think?

For those New Age systems and beliefs that are purported to have real effects, but have not yet been studied using methods that control for chance effects (and related errors), the best we can say is that we do not know whether or not they work. It is as irresponsible for hardnosed skeptics to reject claims out of hand simply because they seem unusual or novel than it is for the New Age practitioners to insist the claims must be true and cannot be a result of observational error. Many New Age claims conflict with established scientific theories. Such scientific theories are linked to massive amounts of high-quality scientific evidence at multiple levels in their own right. The more extreme a New Age claim is, the more extreme evidence is needed to support it, and the more justified scientists are in doubting it. This is not ego-driven scientific authoritarianism; it is the existing scientific observational data and the theories developed from them that the new claim is up against. Still, in untested instances, it remains good practice to empirically test the claims; indeed, it is the only option other than continued ignorance.

Testing claims takes resources, which is exactly why in 1998, the Congress of the United States established a new Institute at the National Institutes of Health (NIH) called the National Institute of Complementary and Alternative Medicine (NCAAM)—later renamed the National Center for Complimentary and Integrative Health. The mission statement of this center is "to define, through rigorous scientific investigation, the usefulness and safety of complementary and alternative medicine interventions and their roles in improving health and health care." As such, claims by New Age practitioners, which are included in "alternative medicine interventions" are not just dismissed, out of hand, as quackery. Rather, they are subjected to testing (using taxpayer dollars) that is designed specifically to control for the types of errors we have been discussing, and to see whether an underlying therapeutic benefit remains after biases and confounders are removed.

If rigorous testing is done and no effect is found, can we then conclude that it is all nonsense? From a scientific point of view, the answer is yes, assuming the trials were done properly, had sufficient statistical power, and were correctly interpreted. In the event that adherents evoke the notion that any testing at all destroys the effect because of negative energy, then science has nothing to say from a deductive logical point of view. However, in such cases it is fair to ask the following question: What is more likely, that an error known to be ubiquitous in human thinking and that has led to all manner of folly over millennia is what is happening again (this is why the effect disappears when methods specifically designed to remove the error are used), or that the very act of questioning whether an effect really exists using such methods somehow negates the effect? This is a hard question to answer when someone is desperate for help and has "experienced" something that works. Ultimately, however, this is the question.

Summary

The ability to predict and control is a fundamental goal of both New Age approaches and science. A clairvoyant, a weather forecaster, a tarot card reader, an epidemiologist tracking COVID-19, a tea-leaf reader, an economist, a palm reader, a climate scientist, a numerologist, and a physician who tests your cholesterol at your annual physical are all doing the same thing. They are using existing theory and understanding to try to predict future events and are generating strategies to intervene. Additional factors are at play (of course), such as the desire to understand and spirituality, but the ability to predict and control is the pragmatic arm of both approaches.

How do we know whether our methods for predicting the future and affecting our condition really work? Regrettably, humans have a great tendency to think things are working when they are not. As discussed in this chapter, we do this by a multipronged assault on the fraction. We distort the fraction by noticing the hits (correct predictions or desired outcomes) and by ignoring the misses. More important, we misperceive the properties of the relevant fraction. We fail to appreciate how big the sample size is. Our attention is drawn to things that seem impossible, when in fact they are highly likely, because we fail to recognize the size of the numerator.

We also move the goal posts, changing the fraction to fit the result we desire, and not what really is. Each time we make these errors, we only reinforce our mistaken beliefs. We feel we know the system is correct because we have seen it work so many times. But 10 million mistaken observations is still no evidence at all.

But some things really do work. How we tell whether a system is working is a fundamental difference between New Age beliefs and science. New Age practitioners know their systems work because they have seen them work. They have experienced the results firsthand and can corroborate their experience with many others. No attempt is made to address the human tendency to misobserve—experience *is* life. In contrast, science addresses human tendencies to misperceive the world. As cognitive psychology learns more and more about the errors humans tend to make, scientists continue to refine their methods to address such errors.

For those who themselves have experienced results, to be told by a scientist that their experience was not real is one hell of a thing. This is like mansplaining to someone what their life is really like, or more like science-splaining. Moreover, New Age practitioners may not want to be corrected. The experience of the mystery and the magic of their practice may be as important as, or more important than, whether or not things work. One reason for the lack of scrutiny about personal experience in New Age beliefs may be because what is being sought is actually the experience in and of itself—and in New Age approaches, reality is defined as what one experiences. Ironically, New Age practitioners may feel victimized by scientists and skeptics who are trying to protect the practitioner from being victimized. The practitioner has found an experience that is highly meaningful to them, without which their life experience would be worse. The scientist is trying to take that away from them. Scientists and skeptics should probably be more respectful of this.

The world that is external to our minds goes on its own way regardless of what we happen to perceive. From a scientific point of view, the question is this: Do you prefer the comfort of your own misperceptions or would you rather find approaches that do more than just provide the experience of working—but that really work? Even more important, do you want to know whether what you are doing in an effort to help is actually harmful? Finally, do you want to know whether you are being victimized by a charlatan? Although this sounds condescending, it is a real concern.

Preferring the comfort of one's own misperceptions over the real world is not necessarily an irrational choice, depending on what exactly is being sought. It is, however, a guarantee of misunderstanding reality, and it prevents any progress in the ability to actually affect what does occur, other than affecting internal experience.

CHAPTER 9

THE APPEARANCE OF DESIGN IN THE NATURAL WORLD

I t is hard to imagine a bigger question than whether or not a god (or gods) exist, what or who they are, and how that should affect our beliefs, our behavior, and how we live our lives. This question has consumed scholars and laypeople over the ages, and has caused controversy, animus, and outright war. There are those on both sides of the debate who feel they know the answer to this question with absolute and unequivocal certainty. We can safely say, however, that no one has yet "proved" the question one way or the other—at least not in the logical meaning of the word "prove"—and certainly not to the satisfaction of those who hold the opposite view.

Much of belief in the divine comes from faith. This book is not about faith, and so we shall leave faith-based discussions to other forums. A long-standing argument has been made, however, that we can prove the divine based upon probability, which is the focus of this book. The argument is based on the observation that the world has such an amazing inner harmony, that it is so "fine-tuned," that the probability of it just coming into being by natural processes is so small as to be essentially impossible. It is certainly rational to not believe impossible things. So, some other explanation is required, the universe must have been purposefully designed. And, if the universe was designed, then there must be a Designer—or so the argument goes.

Arguments Around Fine-Tuning

To consider the fine-tuning argument, we first should review an analogy that goes back hundreds of years (at least), with similar arguments as far back as antiquity. In his 1802 book entitled *Natural Theology, or Evidences of the Existence and Attributes of the Deity Collected from the Appearances of Nature*, William Paley commented on the seemingly clear and unequivocal appearance of purposeful design throughout nature.[1]

Consider that you are walking through the woods one day enjoying the nature all around you. The trees, the dirt, the rocks are all distributed in a typical haphazard way. But then, you notice an old-style pocket watch on the ground. It has a glass front, allowing you to see all the intricate gears and cogs, ticking away in harmonious unison. This is no less lovely than the rest of nature around you, but it certainly does not seem to be "natural"; clearly, pocket watches do not just occur in nature; they are made by craftspeople.[2] There must have been a watchmaker.[3]

The world is an amazingly intricate system of highly integrated pieces that work together like the mechanics of a precision pocket watch. The mathematical constants of the universe are precise to an astounding degree, and even the smallest deviation would render our universe unstable or at least not able to sustain life as we know it. The world certainly has the appearance of being designed. Just like the pocket watch, the likelihood of the world just happening to be so fine-tuned by accident approaches zero. There must have been a Designer. This has been called the fine-tuning argument.

The fine-tuning argument can be divided into two related, but separate, issues. The first issue is how highly fine-tuned life is. Plants and animals have exquisite fine-tuning to themselves, to each other, and to their environment. Paley focused on this in particular, noting the intricately fine-tuned inner workings of animals. How could this possibly happen by chance alone? The second issue is the fine-tuning of the physical properties of the universe that has allowed it both to be stable and capable of supporting life. Let's take these arguments one at a time, with the following consideration in mind: There is no debate that the world has the appearance of being designed. Instead, we are asking whether this appearance is the result of human misperception.

The Fine-Tuning of Life

Plants would all die without bees to pollinate them and bees would die without nectar from the plant's flowers. This is just one example from an endless array of fine-tuned properties of life. Life on Earth is one massive interdependent web of fine-tuning. This is just the tip of the iceberg, however. Life not only is fine-tuned to other forms of life, but also is fine-tuned to itself at the anatomical, microscopic, and molecular levels. The more modern science learns about the molecular and cellular mechanisms of life, the more obvious fine-tuning becomes, adding ever more evidence to Paley's argument. Specific molecules interact with, modify, and regulate other molecules in networks of eloquent complexity. As a professional molecular biologist, I see this every day and it simply amazes me and always will. In addition, and just as amazing, the fine-tuned argument also extends to how fine-tuned the Earth is to life.

Water is one of the only liquids that expands as it freezes, such that lakes freeze from the top and not the bottom; otherwise, all the fish would die in cold climates in winter. If the atmosphere did not filter out just the right kind of light, the Sun's rays would be lethal, but if the atmosphere did not also let other specific types of light through, then plants could not carry out photosynthesis. Bodies of salt water have just the right salinity for the fish that live in them. If the salt concentrations go up or down by much, then the fish die. The examples go on and on: every detail of the Earth seems to fit the requirements of some form of life.

Those reflecting on the fine-tuning of life often allow for only two possible origins; either life was created by a Designer or it simply came into being at random. If the random occurrence of life is so improbable as to be impossible then the only plausible explanation that remains is the existence of a Designer. This type of logic is correct, assuming that there can be only two explanations. If the only options are explanation A or explanation B, and you can rule out explanation B, then it proves A. This logic does not work, however, unless A and B are the only possible explanations. If we identify even one other explanation (e.g., C), then ruling out B no longer proves A, it just eliminates B. Just such an option C was presented in 1858 by Charles Darwin and Alfred Russell Wallace—that is, evolution by natural selection.[4]

The fine-tuned argument is a statement on probability. Like any probability statement, it can be represented by a fraction—here, that fraction is the highly intricate fine-tuned nature of life being on the top of the fraction (the numerator) and all the endless and infinite other ways that the world could be on the bottom of the fraction (the denominator). It is the odds that matter spontaneously happened to form into a watch versus all the other ways matter could be distributed. The use of the fine-tuned argument against evolution, however, results from a fundamental misunderstanding of evolution.

Evolution by natural selection does not involve a Designer, but neither is it random. True, the raw material that natural selection acts on arises through random mutation, but this does not mean that evolution is an overall random or accidental process. Evolution happens by a specific mechanism that, when fully understood, avoids the problems presented by the fine-tuned argument entirely, as explained in the next section.

A Self-Adjusting Fraction: Why Evolution Converts the Fine-Tuned Properties of Life from a Probabilistic Impossibility to a Certainty

Consider a young married couple who is seeking their first apartment together; it is an exciting time. They are lucky to find a spacious two-bedroom flat with a magnificent view of a picturesque lake. This apartment has a large kitchen with many modern amenities, including a built-in oven, an island with a large range and racks above it from which one can hang pots and pans, a fancy dishwasher, refrigerator and freezer, and a microwave. This apartment also has two bathrooms, an additional room that serves as an office/den, and a bay window with an alcove that has built-in bookshelves. Neither newlywed has ever had their own apartment, they were each living with their parents while they were finishing college, so they had only a few possessions. Luckily, they both just got new jobs, with good income, and could afford to furnish their new apartment.

The couple purchases a new king-size bed for the master bedroom, along with nightstands and a dresser. They measure the living room and have a sectional sofa custom made to fit just right, so that they can enjoy the view out their window but still see the television cabinet they purchased to fit against the other wall. They choose a desk that fits perfectly in the office as well as some wooden filing cabinets to match. Given the fancy kitchen, they started getting into cooking, accumulating many pots and pans that they hung from the pot rack. They purchased a nice collection of wine that they kept in their cooler and enjoyed drinking together. They both love to read and ordered many books to fill their shelves. After they had been living there for a year, they become pregnant; so, they purchase furniture to convert the second bedroom into a nursery; luckily, they have a healthy child nine months later.

Consider if we came upon this couple as an outside observer, knowing nothing about them or their history, but encountering them only in the context of their apartment. Might we not look at them and marvel at how well the apartment was designed for their specific needs? It has just the right number of bedrooms for their family, even with a nursery that fits their furniture and child precisely. It has exactly the right shelf space, inch by inch, for the books they have—not one too few books, not one too many, and all the right size. It has precisely the correct size wine cooler for the bottles of wine they have, down to the exact number. Even the number of pot hooks over the range is identical to the number of pots they have. The living room is exactly the correct space for their sofa, to the inch. Given all of the possible sizes and configurations that an apartment may take, what are the odds that this apartment would be so fine-tuned to its occupants by accident; the odds seem vanishingly small, and as such, the most reasonable conclusion is that a Designer specifically made this apartment for this family.

If we were to place a condition on this story that the family and all their belongings randomly sprung fully formed into existence, then the odds that the apartment would perfectly fit them are vanishingly small. In that case, it would be reasonable to conclude that the family and the apartment could only be so fine-tuned to each other if they were purposefully designed; anything else would simply be too unlikely. If, however, the family could modify itself to fit the apartment over time (as in our story), and we saw only the family and the apartment after the fact, then it would have the appearance of a highly unlikely event of fine-tuning. In actuality, it would have been the inevitable result of the family's adaptation to the apartment. This is the basic view from an evolutionary perspective.

Therefore, we can see that if life sprung forth fully formed, and the world came into being instantly and independently from life, then the odds that the two would match the way they do are so infinitesimal that a Designer is by far the best explanation—anything else would be so unlikely as to seem impossible. In the event that life evolved slowly, adapting to the environment in which it found itself, then fine-tuning is an inevitable property of life itself, because it will auto-tune to its environment. In this case, we do not need to evoke a Designer to explain the fine-tuned nature of life. If life is evolving to fit to the environment in which it finds itself, then the probability of life being fine-tuned becomes 100 percent precisely because life adapts to whatever the world is.

Other life is also a part of the environment, and thus evolution fine-tunes life to itself and to other life-forms. The same applies to the internal molecular harmonies of living things. Needless to say, the environment of the Earth is also changing, and as it does, what is adaptive in life changes with it: life-forms are always evolving to catch up with the changing environment. Normal rates of change (outside things like massive meteors, volcanic eruptions, or the destructive force of humans) are typically slow and life keeps up pretty well. When environmental change is rapid, then mass extinction events occur and new varieties of life emerge, a process no less self-tuning than normal evolution—just messier.

It makes no difference that the young couple was mindfully and purposefully adapting to the apartment through intention and that evolution does so through random variations emerging based on reproductive success. What matters is that any system in which the occupant of an environment adapts to that environment (by whatever mechanism) will have the appearance of a highly fine-tuned circumstance with no Designer required.

When two things exist, and one adapts constantly to the other, then fine-tuning is no longer improbable, it is inevitable. If different UV wavelengths were filtered by the atmosphere, then plants would have evolved mechanisms to perform photosynthesis with the light that was available, and life would have evolved protective mechanisms against the more damaging rays. If the salinity of the oceans was different, then life would have evolved different salt requirements.

If water did not freeze from the top down, then life would have evolved a way to either survive being frozen (as some life-forms on Earth can already do) or a way to get out of the water (as other life-forms on Earth can do).

Those who marvel at the fine-tuning of life might as well sit and marvel at how precisely the concrete in a pool fits around the shape of the water in it, and how amazingly perfectly the water fits the pool, even with twists and turns and small cracks. What are the odds of this happening, and not just for one pool, but for every pool! No, given how precisely the pool fits the shape of the water and the water fits the pool, clearly an advanced intelligence with astounding engineering and precision designed each body of water and each pool to fit each other perfectly, molecule by molecule and atom by atom. Anything else is so improbable as to be absurd.[5]

A detailed exploration of how evolution by natural selection works and why it is counterintuitive to human thinking is outside the scope of this book; however, several excellent works explore these issues.[6] Our main point is focused on the probability argument about the fine-tuned nature of life to itself and the Earth. Evolution is essentially a self-adjusting fraction that guarantees that life is fine-tuned to itself and its environment. Both creation of life by a Designer and evolution by natural selection explain an exquisitely fine-tuned world. As such, the fine-tuned nature of life is no proof of a Designer, and in fact, may be no evidence at all.

Is the Self-Correcting Fraction of Evolution Circular Reasoning?

One criticism of evolution is that its predictions are so vague and nondeterministic that the theory essentially cannot be rejected, relegating it to the same status as a pseudoscience. Evolution predicts that as the environment changes, then new varieties of life will emerge that have adapted to the environment. Evolution, however, cannot predict what will emerge, how fast it will emerge, or what precise characteristics it will have.

Moreover, because randomness gives rise to the genetic variation upon which evolution acts, the same initial conditions may lead to different outcomes each time they occur and with all other things being equal. In other words, all evolution indicates is that something will happen, but it cannot specify what will happen, and therefore anything that happens seems to confirm the theory. Nothing can reject it, making it a circular and self-fulfilling tautology. This interpretation, however, is a misunderstanding of evolution. The fact that evolution does not make highly specific and precise predictions regarding the details of what life emerges does not mean it makes no predictions at all.

The evidence that evolution is currently a driving force of emergence of new biological traits is overwhelming. Before the advent of penicillin as an antibiotic, essentially 100 percent of a number of different varieties of bacteria were killed by penicillin. Only with its widespread and persistent use did strains of penicillin-resistant bacteria emerge. The same has been observed with essentially every other antibiotic that has been introduced, and not only for bacteria but also for larger organisms (such as parasites and insects). Evolution could not predict the exact mechanism of resistance, but it did predict resistance. Had no resistance emerged, to any antibiotic used over time, then this would have been a real problem for evolutionary theory.

Charles Darwin devoted a major portion of his book *On the Origin of Species* to problems with the theory—problems that if they could not be solved would result in rejection of evolution. Overtime, those problems have been solved (based on empirical evidence and increased understanding). A great many things could have rejected the theory of evolution, such as the age of the Earth, the "washing out" effect of genetic traits based on the now obsolete theory of genetic blending, and whether or not genetic adaptation of life to a changing environment was observed going forward. The answers of independent scientific exploration in other fields (e.g. geology, thermodynamics, atomic theory, and molecular genetics) have generated answers that support evolution and ultimately have failed to reject evolutionary theory. The answers could have turned out differently and evolution would then have to be rejected, or at least fundamentally changed, but such has not turned out to be the case so far.

Those who advocate for evolution by natural selection and those who oppose it have many issues of disagreement and debate. The literature is full of extensive discussion of such issues, which are outside the scope of this book—except for the probability-based argument of fine-tuning. That life is so fine-tuned that a Designer is the best explanation, or even the only explanation, is simply not the case. Indeed, and somewhat ironically, evolution predicts the fine-tuned nature of life better than a Designer. Why is this? True, a Designer might have made a universe with fine-tuned life in it, but this does not need to be the case. A Designer might have chosen to make life poorly tuned or to have no life at all. In contrast, over time, evolution by natural selection can only produce fine-tuned life, because it is a self-adjusting fraction. Fine-tuned life is one possible outcome of a Designer, but it is a deducible and necessary logical consequence of evolution. This does not speak, however, to the fine-tuned nature of the non-living world; clearly, evolution by natural selection cannot explain the exquisite fine-tuned physical constants of the universe.

The Fine-Tuned Physical Universe

One can list multiple physical properties and constants in the universe. If any of them deviated from their actual values, even a little, then the universe would not be stable let alone capable of supporting life as we know it. For the purposes of this discussion, let's grant that this is a correct and accurate statement. Let us also assume that even this is an underestimate of the fine-tuned nature of our universe. It is likely that scientists have not yet discovered myriad other properties and constants. This adds up to an extremely, almost unimaginably, unlikely universe. So, we are back to square one in the fine-tuned debate. The odds that our current universe should come into being by chance alone, both stable and capable of supporting life without a Designer, is so vanishingly small that it is essentially impossible.

The famous and highly accomplished physicist and mathematician, Roger Penrose, has estimated that for our universe to exist, then the precision of the original phase-space volume of the universe would have to be 1 raised to the power of 10, raised again to the power of 123.[7] In his words:

> This now tells us how precise the Creator's aim must have been: namely to an accuracy of one part in $10^{10^{123}}$. This is an extraordinary figure. One could not possibly even *write the number down* in full, in the ordinary denary notation: it would be a '1' followed by 10^{123} successive '0's! Even if we were to write a '0' on each separate proton and on each separate neutron in the entire universe—and we could throw in all the other particles as well for good measure—we should fall far short of writing down the figure needed.[8]

In other words, the odds are so unlikely, that there are too few particles in the entire universe upon which to write down the number. Now those are *long* odds indeed! Thus, to speculate that the universe just happened at random, is about as close to impossible as one can get. In the words of famous astrophysicist Fred Hoyle:

> "Some super-calculating intellect must have designed the properties of the carbon atom, otherwise the chance of my finding such an atom through the blind forces of nature would be utterly minuscule." A commonsense interpretation of the facts suggests that a super intellect has monkeyed with physics, as well as with chemistry and biology, and that there are no blind forces worth speaking about in nature. The numbers one calculates from the facts seem to me so overwhelming as to put this conclusion almost beyond question.[9]

A large number of accomplished scholars (from theologians to physicists) accept the fine-tuning argument as unequivocal evidence of the necessity of a Designer. However, even highly accomplished scholars are human. Because the fine-tuned argument is based on probability, then issues of how humans perceive probability are essential.

Analogous to how evolution by natural selection coverts the fine-tuned nature of life from an impossibility to a certainty, even in the absence of a Designer, another argument converts the impossibility of the fine-tuned physical universe that we observe into a certainty, even in the absence of a Designer. This argument has been called the anthropic principle.

The Anthropic Principle

During World War II, Allied engineers wanted to reinforce the armor on bombers flying treacherous missions over enemy territory. Because of the weight of the armor, the engineers needed to selectively reinforce only the most vulnerable part of the planes. This should have been a straightforward exercise. Examine the planes that returned from missions, find the parts of the planes with the most damage, and then add armor to those areas. The Statistical Research Group at Columbia University, who were analyzing this problem, had a different solution. Analysis headed up by mathematician Abraham Wald suggested just the opposite—reinforce the planes only in areas that sustained the least damaged.

Leave it to a bunch of ivory tower academics with no real-world experience to come up with a stupid idea like that. It defied common sense. When engineers inspect bridges, and they find stress fractures in the metal of certain areas, those are the areas that need to be repaired and reinforced. Would it make any sense to reinforce the areas that had no damage at all and leave the stress fractures alone? Try defending that to the court of inquiry after the bridge collapses during rush hour. Why would any sane person choose to only reinforce the parts of planes that took the least damage and to ignore the parts that were most damaged?

By focusing on the areas of the planes that almost never had damage, Wald was isolating the most vulnerable part, the striking of which would most likely lead to it crashing. In the case of the bridge, all bridges were being examined. The only planes being examined were those that survived their missions and made it back to base. No data were available on the planes that were destroyed by enemy fire; they never returned. Wald reasoned that the part of the plane that could be damaged the most without causing the plane to crash would have the most hits in planes that made it back to base. Any area that was really vulnerable, that when hit would easily destroy the plane, should have the least damage in the planes that returned (i.e., those that managed to survive the missions).[10] Wald's groundbreaking analysis and important counterintuitive insights are essential to understanding what is called the "survivorship bias."

What does all this have to do with the fine-tuned universe? Just as only planes that survive the mission can be observed by engineers, only universes that are stable and can sustain life can be observed by living things. Universes that are physically unstable would cease to exist. Any stable universes that came into being would "exist," but if they could not sustain life, then no one could ever know they were there. In universes in which creatures exist who are debating the origins of their universe, the odds of a stable universe that can support life are 100 percent. If you interviewed 100 people who had played Russian roulette, 100 percent of them would rate themselves as very lucky. In other words, the exceptional fined-tuned nature of the universe no longer needs an explanation as it is no longer highly improbably: it is now a certainty. This is called the anthropic principle.[11]

The anthropic principle has been criticized as an oversimplistic fallacy that changes the question being asked.[12] As explained by Stephen C. Meyer, philosopher John Leslie pointed out that advocates of the anthropic principle

> focus on the wrong phenomenon of interest. They think that what needs to be explained (or explained away) is why *we observe* a universe consistent with our existence. It's true that such an observation is not surprising. What needs explanation, though, is what caused the fine tuning of the universe in the first place—not our later observation of it.[13]

In other words, it may be true that we should not be surprised that we live in a universe that can sustain life. This is the only type of universe we could live in. Rather, we should be surprised that we (and our particular universe) exist at all. The fact that we are observing our universe does not alter that the odds of our universe being as fine-tuned as it is remains so astoundingly small as to approach being impossible. It remains rational not to believe impossible things. For this reason, Meyer (and many others) find that a Designer is the only reasonable explanation.

The Certainty of Impossible Accidents

Importantly, the question (as Meyer states it) is a question of cause: "What caused the fine-tuning of the universe in the first place?"[14] This is an excellent question, but the use of the word "caused" presupposes that the universe was *caused* to be fine-tuned (either by a Designer, a naturalistic mechanism, or even something else we have not conceived of yet). This seems to be a reasonable assumption: if our universe was not caused to be fine-tuned, then why is it so?

Like the universe, each of us as individual humans can be viewed as an incredibly unlikely event. True, there are far more possible universes than possible people. Still, the average ejaculate has about 150 million sperm (the average male makes about 500 billion sperm in a lifetime).[15] The average female is born with one to two million eggs in her ovaries, only about 400 of which are ever released during ovulation. What are the odds that the one particular sperm that led to you (out of the 500 billion your father will make in his life) would meet that particular egg (out of one to two million) from your mother?

We cannot stop with the odds of one sperm from your father meeting one egg from your mother at one particular moment and to the exclusion of all other sperm and eggs. The same goes for your grandparents on both sides, all eight of your great grandparents, all 16 of your great-great-grandparents, and so on and so on back to the beginning (whenever that was). Moreover, this example refers only to the odds of conception. What about the odds that any of your breeding ancestors ever lived long enough to reproduce, ever actually met the person with whom they did reproduce, and forget the odds of convincing the partner to engage in the act?

By the time any of us is born, we are already an unimaginably improbable event, but that does not mean we are impossible. After all, we are here. If you are reading this, then you are presumably a person who exists.[16] Of all the possible humans you could have been, the odds of you being exactly as you are is close to zero. The immediate cause of your existence is that your parents bred and you were born—but this is not the cause of why you are the specific version of human you are. We do not demand an explanation for why you inherited exactly the genetics you did or have the specific traits you have. You can only be a single human, and as such, you can only have a single set of genetics and traits. There is no mystery here.

If we assume only one universe (more on this later), then whatever one universe comes into existence will be so unlikely as to be close to impossible. This can be couched in a variation of the lottery fallacy described in chapter 7. Before the Powerball lottery is drawn, any of the 292 million possible number combinations could be drawn; each is equally improbable. A drawing will occur, however, and one of them (and only one of them) will be the winning combination. Although it is equally improbable that any number combination will be drawn, it is even less probable that no number combination will be drawn. No matter what combination is drawn, a highly improbable event is guaranteed, and therefore, no other explanation is needed when it occurs.

What if the universe really did come about by accident? True, the odds of our universe having the specific fine-tuned properties it has are astoundingly small. But the odds of whatever one universe would exist having no properties are zero. If every version of the universe is equally unlikely, then any universe that will be (or even could be) would be unimaginably improbable. The probability is the same for constants that prohibit any universe from ever coming to be in the first place. In this light, the fine-tuned nature of our universe needs no explanation at all—just as you do not need to explain why you have the specific human traits that you have or why certain numbers were the winning Powerball combination this week.

Mountain Carvings and Rubble Below: Why Our Everyday Experience Is Not Relevant to Our Universal Speculations

The driving question behind fine-tuned arguments is how a universe as unlikely as ours possibly could come to be without some intervention from a Designer. We have been exploring the notion that while our universe is amazingly unlikely, any universe would be equally unlikely. So nothing is particularly in need of explanation. The unlikeliness of our universe is not special; it is inevitable and it would be found in any universe.

Some people think, however, that the existence of our particular universe needs to be explained. Although every universe may be equally unlikely, not every universe has the special properties ours does. Of course, every universe would have some special properties particular to that version of the universe. So why do the special properties of our universe need to be explained?

William Dembski, a mathematician and philosopher, explains this using a now-classic example comparing the placement of stones in a garden.

> In one instance the stones spell "Welcome to Wales by British Railways," in the other they appear randomly strewn. In both instances the precise arrangement of stones is vastly improbable. Indeed, any given arrangement of stones is but one of an almost infinite number of possible arrangements. Nevertheless, arrangements of stones that spell coherent English sentences form but a minuscule proportion of the total possible arrangements of stones. The improbability of such arrangements is not properly referred to chance.[17]

Dembski goes on to clearly acknowledge that "everything conforms to some pattern or other—even a random arrangement of stones. The crucial question, therefore, is whether an arrangement of stones conforms to the right sort of pattern to eliminate chance." But how can there be a "right" sort of pattern and a "wrong" sort of pattern? Dembski explains that humans have the ability to recognize patterns that indicate an intelligence behind them and sets out specific criteria for doing so.[18]

Stephen Meyer explains Dembski's position by an analogy focusing on Mount Rushmore: the iconic carving of the faces of four U.S. presidents into a mountainside in South Dakota. The monument was painstakingly sculpted by 400 workers over a period of 14 years, subsequent to the unlawful seizing of the land by the United States from the Lakota Nation.[19] Meyer points out:

If you look at that famous mountain you will quickly recognize the faces of the American presidents inscribed there as the product of intelligent activity. Why? . . . the faces on the mountain qualify as extremely improbable structures, since they contain many detailed features that natural processes do not generally produce. Certainly, wind and erosion, for example, would be unlikely to produce the recognizable faces of Washington, Jefferson, Lincoln, and Roosevelt. . . . the precise arrangement of the rocks at the bottom of the mountain also represents an extremely improbable configuration, especially when one considers all the other possible ways those rocks might have settled.[20]

The point Meyer is making, and quite correctly so, is that while both the faces in the mountain and the rubble at the bottom are identically unlikely configurations of matter, we assign an intelligent and purposeful source to the former but not the latter. Why do we do this? Meyer explains:

The answer is the presence of a special kind of pattern . . . we see a shape or pattern that *matches* one we know from independent experience, namely, from seeing the human face and even the specific faces of the presidents on money or in history books . . . intelligent agents recognize intelligent activity whenever they observe a highly improbable object or event that also matches an independently recognizable or meaningful pattern. The pile of stones at the bottom of the cliff does not form such a pattern, but the faces on the mountain do.[21]

Meyer is quite correct in his assertions, and one must pay them due respect. Indeed, the very type of pattern recognition he is describing would be highly adaptive in any evolutionary environment. If one is wandering around a forest, and sees a fire pit and a tent, one can infer that a human has been there, and may still be nearby, or even may be sleeping in the tent. Being able to tell when an intelligent being has been, or still is, present offers a significant advantage over the alternative of having no ability to predict the presence of others.

An essential component of Meyer's argument is evident in his words: "we see a shape or pattern that *matches* one we know from independent experience." Herein lies the problem with the argument. Our experience, at least thus far, is particular to properties of intelligent agents (or their absence) on Earth. We have a lot of experience about how mountains and rock rubble tend to look when no one has acted on them. Likewise, we have a lot of experience about what stone sculptures made by intelligent agents (in this case, humans) look like.

We must ask ourselves, how much experience do we actually have comparing a vast number of different universes that were made by a Designer with those that came into existence by natural forces without a Designer? The answer, or course, is no experience whatsoever—not even a single universe, because we do not know the origin of our own. The relevance of our experience to other circumstances rests entirely on the other circumstances having similar properties to that which we have experienced. We have no basis, whatsoever, to suspect that the rules of rock carving on Earth are similar to rules of universe creation.

When we do not have experience-based metrics to guide us about how we evaluate a situation, then theory and understanding can be helpful. In this case, however, we have zero understanding of the rules behind universe creation (in general) and clearly we struggle to define the process by which our own universe came into being. We do not even know whether our universe *did* come into being. True, our universe is here, and it seems natural to us that we should ask where it came from. But what if our universe is simply eternal, as has been held both by multiple theologies and philosophers?

Of course, none of this is evidence against a Designer having created the universe; that remains a formal possibility. The fact that disproving a Designer's involvement is a logical impossibility does not, in of itself, decrease the likelihood of such an explanation. The analysis developed in this section, however, does eliminate the requirement for invoking a Designer to explain the universe because of probability-based fine-tuning arguments. So, does a Designer remain the most likely explanation?

Although we do not have any experience around creation of universes, we do have a great deal of experience in how humans tend to misperceive things they do not understand. Humans have a profound tendency to see mindful action where it does not exist. Humans have a "theory of mind" by which we imagine intelligences in natural settings where they do not occur.[22] We have the capacity to perceive conspiracies where none exist and dream all kind of purposeful acts behind random events. We also know that humans have a strong tendency to misperceive probability. We do not like the idea of things happening accidentally and feel that there must be reasons behind what occurs. This is an issue of human aesthetics and intuition, which can frequently be wrong. So, if we are focusing on probability-based arguments, what is more probable? That an invisible Designer created the universe with us in it or that we are simply misperceiving probability and assigning intelligent causes where none exist, as humans have repeatedly done throughout our history?

The Multiverse Hypothesis

It should be clear that the fine-tuning debate is a struggle to explain how such an improbable universe as our own came to be. If the universe was designed, then there is no mystery. Likewise, if we are misperceiving the probability, then we have nothing to explain. A third resolution to the problem is to modify the fraction through expanding the numerator so as to increase the probability. This can be done by positing the existence of multiple universes.

The multiverse hypothesis, as this is called, suggests that humans are analyzing the wrong fraction—much like the lottery fallacy described in chapter 7. The top of the fraction of our amazingly small probability (only one universe) is expanded. Taken to an extreme, if all possible universes existed, and the inhabitants of any one universe were unaware of the other universes, then every life-form would think its universe was unique and amazingly unlikely when in reality, each universe was a certainty. If every possible stable universe that can exist does exist, then the numerator equals the denominator, and the odds are 100 percent. We, however, can only see one version of the fraction (with one universe as the numerator). Thus, it looks like we live in a highly improbable world.

With all due respect to those who support the multiverse hypothesis, the existence of a multiverse is a fairly radical claim. What justification supports such a proposition? The motivation for positing the multiverse is clear. It provides an alternative explanation for why the universe is so fine-tuned. Positing an unobserved entity to reconcile a paradox is nothing new. Even in the hard-core sciences, this happens all the time. Scientists are adept at imagining unobserved causes of observable effects to advance new theories. Moreover, these causes often are not directly observable, and their existence can only be inferred from the observable effects they cause. At least in the sciences, however, it is typically not enough to suggest the existence of a previously unappreciated thing because it can explain some component of observation; rather, positing the new entity must lead to some new prediction that can be tested. If that prediction is not observed, all things being equal, then the hypothesis should be rejected—or at least modified to reconcile the contradiction caused by the disconfirming evidence.

So, is there an experiment we can conduct to seek evidence to refute or support the existence of the multiverse? Many physicists believe the current answer to this question is "no." That said, many theories we now hold as true could not be tested when they were first proposed, because the full implications of the theory were not yet appreciated or the technologies to test them did not exist. The history of science is that as theories mature, and intersect with other theories, and technologies advance, then testable predictions are sometimes generated. Still, the historical wastebins of science are full of theories that never made any testable predictions and thus were discarded. For the multiverse, time will tell. This does not mean, however, that evidence to support the notion of a multiverse is completely lacking.

An indirect way to test a theory is to see whether it intersects with other theories, which themselves are grounded in observation. For example, certain theoretical outcomes of the big bang theory predict other universes, and the big bang theory has given rise to predictions that ultimately were tested and held up to scrutiny. The prediction of cosmic microwave background radiation by the big bang was discovered by Arno Penzias and Robert Wilson. In this case, confirmation bias was likely not at play, because Penzias and Wilson were not thinking about the origins of the universe. Rather, they were busy trying to invent a new communication system at Bell Labs and were desperately trying to get rid of the background signal. They realized they could not because the signal actually was distributed throughout the universe.

The multiverse is part of some versions of the big bang theory, and the big bang theory has held up to some empirical scrutiny. Thus, by proxy, multiverses are linked to some empirical support. Is this evidence for a multiverse? Yes, it is some evidence, but not much and it is certainly indirect. Perhaps of greater concern is the fact that the big bang theory predicts that such multiverses are so far away we could never observe them, and they are moving even farther away at incredible speeds.

Thus, directly testing the multiverse hypothesis does not seem likely. It is for this reason that Paul Davies has stated that "the multiverse theory hovers on the borderline between science and fantasy."[23] It is also for this reason that many scientists do not view the multiverse hypothesis as a scientific hypothesis. Because it cannot be tested, it is not science; however, this in no way demonstrates that it is not true. To the contrary, it guarantees direct evidence can never be generated to reject the hypothesis, but nor can direct evidence support it, at least not by scientific approaches. Respectfully, the hypothesis of a Designer is in the same boat. It explains the world we observe, but it ultimately is untestable. Thus, while interesting, the multiverse hypothesis remains a weak explanation of the fine-tuned universe.

You Can't Explain Everything So There Must Be a Designer of the Universe

We do not know whether rules govern the formation of the universe. For all we know, our universe is the only possible universe. Likewise, we do not know that the only two options are creation by a Designer or spontaneous coming into being. Notice that when the fine-tuned nature of the universe is used as an argument for a Designer, the logic is that without another plausible explanation, then we must have a Designer—it is the only option remaining. This is a highly useful and common type of reasoning called inference to the best explanation.[24] This type of reasoning suffers one major flaw (i.e., the fallacy of limited hypotheses): inference to the best explanation can never achieve proof of an explanation unless the number of possible explanations can be limited, and there is no basis to limit potential theories of the universe.

In an endless number of murder mysteries, the brilliant detective catches the killer by ruling out all the possible suspects, except one, who must then be guilty. But imagine a mystery with an infinite number of suspects. The history of science is littered with the fallacy of limited hypotheses, over and over again. For 300 years, physicists argued whether light was a wave or a particle—assuming those were the only two options. Often, those favoring one hypothesis "proved" it by rejecting the other option, leaving their favored explanation as the only one left. This logic only works, however, if there can only be two options. Our best current understanding is that light is neither a wave nor a particle but it is some other thing we do not have an analogy for in normal experience. Both leading hypotheses were incorrect—the answer is some other explanation.

Just because a Designer cannot be proved does not mean it is not the correct explanation. The absence of evidence is not the evidence of absence. At the same time, even if we reject all explanations other than a Designer, this is not logical support for a Designer unless we limit the number of possible explanations—and we have no justification for such a limit. How many other explanations are there that humans have not yet thought of? How many explanations are there that humans are incapable of understanding or conceiving? The limits of human cognition do not limit the nature of the universe, just what we are able to consider. Finally, as explored in this chapter, the puzzle of a fine-tuned universe may be no puzzle at all—just a human misperception of probability.

Lastly, I feel it is important to consider what it would mean if one swept away all the arguments presented in this chapter and simply acknowledged that the universe is so highly improbable that it could not have come about on its own. Therefore, there must have been a Designer. One must then ask, but where did the Designer come from? Did the Designer have a Designer as well? If so, then who Designed that Designer? This argument is often answered by stating that the Designer is eternal, with no beginning or end, and has thus simply always been. However, in this case, one is trading the improbability of something as wondrous as our universe simply coming into being for the improbability of something as wondrous as the Designer simply coming into being. As explained by John Allen Paulos, "If a certain entity is very complex and it's deemed extraordinarily unlikely that such complexity would have arisen by itself, then what is explained by attributing the entity's unlikely complexity to an even more complex and even more unlikely source?"[25] So, even if we could reject the universe coming into being on its own, through probability-based fine-tuning arguments, we could not then justify the explanation of a Designer as a better alternative, as it suffers the very same problems of improbability.

Summary

It is rational to believe things that are probably true and to discount things that are highly improbable. Indeed, if something is improbable enough, it can be considered impossible for practical purposes. Of all the possible universes that could be, the odds that our particular universe would come to be are unimaginably small. Yet here we are. Of all the possible ways that life could exist, the odds that it would be so intricately fine-tuned to itself and the world around it, are also unimaginably small. These odds would be made more likely, or even certain, if a Designer had made the universe and the life in it. However, these odds also would be made more likely, or even certain, if we misperceived the probability and if the fraction adjusted itself to 100 percent.

Regarding the fine-tuned nature of life, evolution by natural selection adjusts the fraction to 100 percent—life tunes itself no less than water conforms to the shape of a pool. If the shape of the pool changes, the water adapts to the new shape. With regards to the properties of the universe, one can make the fraction 100 percent by positing a multiverse, but it is unclear that we have (or ever will have) direct evidence of a multiverse. More compelling is that if a life-form has sufficient intelligence to ponder the universe it is living in, then there is a 100 percent chance that it is living in a stable universe that can support life. This anthropic principle is an example of the survivorship bias, as with planes returning to the base in World War II, and it changes the probability of fine-tuning to 100 percent.

Finally, with regards to the fine-tuned physical properties of the universe, it is unclear that there is anything to explain. Regardless of how unlikely any given universe is to exist, if there is just one universe, then whatever form it takes will be equally unlikely. This is just a human misperception of probability. The fact that the universe has the "appearance of being designed" is not in question, but rather human experience in what a designed universe looks like is zero, which makes the appearance to humans hold little value.

This chapter does not argue about the existence of a Designer, or lack thereof, and whether or not the world or life were created. Rather, this chapter illustrates that the fine-tuned argument is fundamentally an argument about probability. As such, how humans understand and misunderstand probability is highly relevant to this debate.

CHAPTER 10

THE HARD SCIENCES

S cientists use specific methods and approaches to decrease errors in observation of the natural world, including errors of misperceiving probability, rates, and frequencies. As explored in chapter 8, this approach is quite distinct from other systems of belief that place a premium on individual experience.

When someone witnesses their personal experience with the divine to other members of a religious congregation, their experience is not typically subjected to a statistical analysis to verify whether it was simply a chance occurrence. It certainly may be doubted or even rejected if it is too extreme or varies too much from the norms of spiritual experience for the group in question. However, experiences are not formally tested by methods meant to compensate for human observational error. One does not typically see a Catholic priest testing whether the perceived benefit of taking communion is "real" by randomizing the congregation into two separate groups, one of which is given consecrated communion wafers and the other of which is given a placebo (i.e., unconsecrated wafers that are indistinguishable from consecrated ones).

In contrast, the maturation of scientific methods has made great progress in decreasing the problem of chance effects and probability. Regrettably, the problem persists in insidious ways, however, and continues to pop up in new and unanticipated areas.

Statistics as a Tool to Mitigate the Problem of Chance Effects

In the early 1900s, a number of brilliant mathematicians began to develop statistical tools to assess the likelihood that differences between two groups reflected a "real" difference versus being chance effects. These tools were developed, part and parcel, with a growing understanding of probability theory, how chance occurrences really happen, and what "random" looks like as opposed to what humans think it looks like.[1]

Consider, for example, if a new drug is being evaluated to treat a disease. A number of patients with the illness in question are enrolled in a study and are assigned either to a group that gets the new drug or a group that does not. If the drug works, then the group getting the drug should have less severe disease than the group not getting the drug. Such studies have all kinds of potential bias, and modern methods of clinical trial design have matured around the issue of mitigating (if not eliminating) such biases.

First, the patients are "randomized" in an attempt to make every variable identical between the two groups, other than receiving the drug. Analysis is done to see how well the randomization worked, such as assessing how similar the groups are with respect to age, sex, ethnic background, and disease severity. Depending on the disease being studied, other factors may be checked, such as diet, alcohol consumption, smoking habits, other illnesses, other medications, and family history. One can seldom (if ever) get complete parity despite randomization, and there are always some differences between the groups, even if only in unmonitored variables. The goal, however, is to get as close as possible to the only difference between the groups being receiving the drug or not.

The group not getting the drug will get a "placebo," which in an ideal world is indistinguishable from the drug being tested.[2] This is to ensure that any benefit from the drug is not due to patients feeling better simply because they know they are receiving a treatment (known as the "placebo effect"). The placebo effect is a very real thing: in and of itself, it can be of tremendous clinical value—a benefit sadly dismissed by many as being "not real." That said, by comparing the treatment group with a placebo group, effects other than placebo effects can be isolated and evaluated.

Ideally, neither the health-care provider nor the patients know which group is getting the drug being tested and which group is getting the placebo (called a double-blinded study). This is done to avoid introducing inadvertent differences other than the drug (e.g., the health-care providers may act differently toward one group or the other) and also to avoid confirmation bias by either the researchers or the patients in the form of interpreting the signs, symptoms, and progression of the disease differently in one group versus another.

Of course, the nature of the treatment and the disease being studied makes it more or less prone to such biases and more or less suitable for bias mitigation.

For example, a drug designed to decrease a subjective symptom during a chronic illness (e.g., feelings of fatigue or sadness) is more vulnerable to bias than an outcome that can be measured through objective instrumentation (e.g., measuring cholesterol in the blood).[3] Clearly, if one is comparing a treatment for acute trauma with the outcome being survival or death, interpreting the outcomes faces less subjectivity.

In some cases, a placebo or blinding is not feasible from a technical or ethical point of view. If you are comparing open heart surgery with a drug treatment, then you cannot blind the doctor or the patient—both the physicians and patients will know who is undergoing open heart surgery and who is not.[4] Optimal experimental practice, however, entails randomized, controlled, double-blinded studies to the extent possible for a given situation.

For the purposes of the current discussion, let us assume that the perfect study is being carried out, that groups are perfectly randomized, that the treatment is the only variable that differs between the groups, and that there is absolutely no bias. What then is the risk of misinterpreting the outcome of the study? What remains problematic is the noisiness of the real world—that is, the possibility of chance effects. Statistics is a powerful tool to quantify likelihood of chance effects.

In our given study, let's assume that the outcome is survival or death (from the disease) over a one-year period of time. One hundred patients are randomized such that 50 receive the drug and 50 receive placebo. Twenty of those getting the placebo die, whereas only 10 of those getting the drug die. So, although not perfect, the drug has efficacy—it causes a decrease in death at one year, right? Actually, the answer to this question is an unequivocal maybe. But why?

The patients are a population of people with the normal variability found in any population. Even if no therapy was given, some people are going to have more or less severe disease. At one year out, some are going to die, whereas others will still be alive. What if people who were going to have less severe disease anyway wound up at a higher frequency in the group getting the drug, just by chance? Such a result would make it look like the drug had efficacy when, in fact, it did not. The question is not if the group getting the drug really had a better outcome (we are stipulating they did). But was this benefit really due to the drug? Mistaking chance differences for a real effect is often called a "type I error."

Advanced statistical methods can monitor type I errors. Studies are designed with careful attention to the "alpha level," which is the frequency of type I errors given a particular experimental design. One can specify any alpha level one wants and set this as the cutoff for what will be accepted as a "real" result as opposed to a chance difference. In other words, what chances of making a type I error are the researchers willing to accept?

By stating the alpha level upfront, and sticking to it, one protects against "moving the goal post fallacies" after the fact. Having set the alpha level, after a study is complete, one can calculate the probability of any difference that was observed being due to chance (called the p value).[5] Numerous methods can be used to calculate p values, based on the sample size, the distribution of the data, whether the data points are interrelated or independent, the study design, and other factors. The correct method must be used, but assuming it is, then if the p value is less than the alpha, the difference is said to be "statistically significant," and if not, then the findings are said to be "statistically insignificant."

Often, statisticians refer to the case in which the drug has no effect as the "null hypothesis." If the drug really does have an effect, then its effects are not "Null" and one can "reject the null hypothesis." To reject the null hypothesis (a regrettable linguistic double negative), simply means to find an effect—in other words, because there is *not* no effect, there is some effect. So, if using an alpha value of 0.05, then if the p value is less than 0.05, we say the results are "statistically significant," and we reject the null hypothesis (the drug has an effect). If the p value is greater 0.05, then the results are not statistically significant, and we fail to reject the null hypothesis (i.e., the drug does not have an effect). How's that for the use of simple language to make science easily understandable to the lay public? Simply stated, if the p value is less than 0.05, the effect is considered real ($p \leq 0.05$ is less than a 5% chance of a type I error, or 1 in 20).

Although powerful, this approach is somewhat arbitrary (e.g., we picked 0.05). Actually, 0.05 is the typical gold standard of most fields, but it is still an arbitrary number that people happen to agree on, mostly.[6] There is nothing fundamental about allowing an error 1 out of every 20 times; however, the cutoff for approval has to be set somewhere to avoid moving the goal posts. Statistics can only quantify our uncertainty, not eliminate it.

Statistics also can be used upfront to tell us how large a study needs to be to decrease uncertainty to a particular level. This is often called a power analysis. Basically, by knowing how large an effect would be meaningful (e.g., how much improvement would a drug need to give to be worth taking) and what likelihood of making a type I error is acceptable, one can determine how many subjects need to be in a study. Of course, research studies consume massive resources. We could demand alpha levels that are very low and apply our resources to the development of many fewer new therapies, but with fewer type I errors. Conversely, we could use our limited resources to develop more therapies but accept higher rates of error. It is a balancing act between what rates of error we are willing to accept versus how much research we can perform and how many things we can test—and, perhaps most important, the ethics of the risk of exposing human subjects to research studies versus the risk of approving drugs that don't really work.[7]

Hacking Your Way to Bias

Scientists often wield statistical tools effectively, but they do so imperfectly. The human tendency toward errors regarding frequencies and probabilities is so strong that it can drive even well-trained scientists to inadvertently pervert statistics to bring about the very kind of errors that the statistics are designed to mitigate. Scientists are incentivized to do so by the way science is supported and carried out, as we shall explore. This is not to suggest that scientists intentionally misuse statistics (although this does occur on occasion). Rather, scientists are human and subject to the foibles of human cognition, such as forms of confirmation bias that invade scientific research despite efforts to keep them out.

The main currency of scientific findings is publication in journals. Journals, however, are selective in what they publish, holding authors to strict standards. Usually, submitted findings are subjected to "peer review"—a process in which other scientists (presumably experts in the field) assess the suitability of the findings for publication. Criteria for acceptance include how much the findings advance the field and contribute to knowledge, but perhaps more important, the scientific rigor of the findings is thoroughly evaluated. The p value of observations is one of the metrics of scientific rigor that often is heavily weighted in the peer-review determination. A p value of 0.05 is currently the gold standard for all manner of research, from basic studies of molecules or cells to whole animal biology, to human clinical trials on new therapies.

Scientists are highly scrutinized according to the number of papers they publish and the prestige of the journals that print them. This can affect the scientist's career in multiple ways, including grant funding, salary and promotion, preeminence in professional societies, and chances to speak in public forums. This means that scientists are highly incentivized and strongly motivated for the results of their studies to be statistically significant (e.g., to have low p values—without which they cannot easily publish.

Sadly, but predictably, the tools of rigor cause problems as well as solving them. The p value becomes a coveted thing that scientists "seek" rather than an objective instrument of evaluating chance effects. In the words of Gary Smith, a statistically significant p value becomes "an odd religion that researchers worship almost blindly."[8] The intense emphasis placed on p values by journals and scientists creates problems at several levels and by different mechanisms.

The regrettable reality is that the p value tends to become the goal, rather than serving as a measure of the actual goal (i.e., high-quality science with the ability to quantify, if not mitigate, uncertainty). This is a manifestation of what is called Campbell's law, named after Donald T. Campbell, the psychologist who described this effect. Campbell's law occurs when a metric itself becomes the primary goal rather than the effect the metric was designed to measure. In his highly amusing and insightful book, *The Tyranny of Metrics*, Jerry Z. Muller goes into deep analytic detail of how the effects of Campbell's law damage scientific pursuits.[9]

Highly important to the current discussion, the tendency of journals to publish findings that have low p values, but not studies that have higher p values, is an error of representing frequency: it is changing the fraction. The scientific communities are blinded to the number of studies that are carried out (the denominator). Let us consider a situation in which 20 different scientists around the world carry out a similar study to test the same hypothesis (e.g., infection with some virus (virus-x) is associated with arthritis). If the hypothesis is correct, then we should observe a higher rate of virus-x infection in people who have arthritis than in people who do not (all other things being equal). In this case, let's assume that the hypothesis is incorrect: no such association between virus-x and arthritis exists. By chance alone, 1 of the 20 investigators will find virus-x present at a higher level in patients with arthritis than in those without arthritis, with a p value equal to or less than 0.05.

If every investigator submitted their findings for publication, then the one study with a low p value would have a much better chance of being published than the others. This has been termed "publication bias" and is a serious issue in science, probably doing far more damage than is generally appreciated. Importantly, judging a report based on the quality of the data, the rigor of the methods and approach, or the validity of the interpretation is not publication bias. Peer review is an essential gatekeeper of the quality of scientific knowledge claims, and failing to hold scientists to high standards of rigor before publishing would be a dereliction of duty. Publication bias persists, however, even having stipulated that all papers being evaluated have 100 percent rigor and are perfectly performed science. In this case, we have bias solely on the statistical significance of the findings.

So, where is the harm? Why should scientific journals fill their pages with "insignificant" findings—isn't it good and appropriate to focus on the significant? We have to pay attention to the meaning of the word "significant." We are not talking about publishing questions of different importance. No one would fault a journal for preferring to publish that a new anti-cancer drug works over the question of whether or not Scandinavian muskrats can taste the extract of the bark from Brazilian rubber trees. Rather, in this case, we are referring to separate studies asking the same question, with the same methods, and the same rigor—it is just that one has a p value below 0.05 and the others do not. The term significance refers only to "statistical significance."

Preferentially publishing studies that are "statistically significant" over those that are not, results in the selective publication of findings that are "positive" and confirm a hypothesis. At the same time, findings that are "negative"— those that reject a hypothesis—are seriously neglected. Rejecting a hypothesis is just as useful as a supporting one, and arguably it is much more useful, because it is of greater deductive logical utility. Findings that reject (e.g., find no effect), however, are often ignored. Moreover, once a publication finds a statistically significant difference, then even if a follow-up study shows no difference, it is typically difficult to get published in a journal of the same caliber, if at all. Equally important is that knowing this barrier to publication, those whose studies had a p value higher than 0.05 (not statistically significant) may never take the time to even write the paper and submit it (called the "file drawer effect").

Thus, publication bias creates an ignorance to how many times studies are done. If one does a study only once and gets a p value less than 0.05, that is of reasonable significance. If, however, one does a study 20 times and gets a p value of less than 0.05 in only one of the 20 studies, then this is what is predicted by chance alone when the measured effect is not real. Regrettably, because of the publication bias and the file drawer effect, a field may do a study 20 times but only report the single instance in which the p value was less than 0.05, leaving the other 19 trials invisible to the field. More commonly, some of the negative studies would be published (albeit in less prestigious journals). This underreporting of the negative studies still exaggerates the significance of the positive study—in other words, ignoring the denominator of the fraction. Sadly, the publication bias and file drawer effects cause exactly the problem that p values were designed to mitigate.

One of the great strengths of science is that it is ultimately self-correcting; even when errors do occur, they do not hold up over time. However, this depends on ongoing study—errors cannot be corrected if no one is investigating them. Knowing of the publication bias toward novel positive findings, scientists are less likely to embark on an effort to retest a previous report of an association. If their studies find the same thing, then it is "me too" science; conversely, if they find the opposite, then publication bias works against them. Either way, their careers and resources for research are likely to be lesser for the effort. Thus, publication bias not only blinds fields to the number of times a study has been carried out but also sometimes prevents follow-up studies from being performed—not just ignoring the denominator but *preventing* the denominator.

Regrettably, the depth of the problem goes much deeper than the direct effects of publication bias. It has been argued that the cutoff of a p value of less than 0.05 has resulted in methodological changes leading to wholesale scientific distortion. This occurs when scientists evaluate a set of data from multiple angles, looking for the associations that have p values less than 0.05. Why is this wrong? Isn't it necessary to mine data to find the significant associations? Yes, the entire point of p values is to allow science to do precisely that. What happens, however, is that scientists wind up analyzing data and changing study design after the fact (or after it is already in progress) with the goal of finding conditions in which p values are low. This is like having a big monitor on the wall showing the real time p value as it evolves, and the scientists play with the study design while staring at the monitor. Whatever makes the p value go down, they pay attention to; whatever makes the p value go up, they ignore.

The problem with this has been described in terms of researchers having too many "degrees of freedom," such as how much data should be collected, what data should be excluded, how conditions should be combined, and how things should be compared. In other words, investigators seek conditions under which a calculated p value drops below the coveted threshold of 0.05. A computer simulation of this process demonstrated that false positive rates (i.e., type I errors) jump as high as 61 percent with only four different degrees of freedom (in this case, choosing between two different dependent variables, being able to add more observations if an initial result is not significant, being able to switch conditions of gender of subjects, and being able to drop one of the above three conditions or to combine them).[10] This example is somewhat contrived and certainly artificial, but it illustrates the point with great potency.

How is this a form of misperceiving the fraction? It is analogous to the lottery fallacy and what we discussed earlier about New Age beliefs and fortune telling (chapters 7 and 8), another example of increasing the numerator of the aggregate fraction. The p value determination is relevant to assessing a limited number of hypotheses (or, in some cases, a single hypothesis). By adjusting many different parameters looking for a p value of less than 0.05, one is massively increasing the number of conditions being studied and effectively testing many different hypotheses. Instead of running a single experiment and finding something that would happen only by chance 1 out of every 20 times ($p = 0.05$), it is like running 20 experiments and finding something that happens by chance 1 out of 20 times, and then only reporting the one time it happened. Clearly, a 61 percent rate of error is a far cry from the generally accepted 5 percent error rate. This throws the whole notion of statistical significance into a very different light, and not a favorable one at that.

These research tendencies have been called "data dredging," "p-hacking," and "inflation bias" and can take multiple forms in addition to what was modeled earlier: selective reporting, dropping outliers during analysis, looking at data partway through a study to decide whether or not to continue, or simply gathering data until a statistically significant result is found and then stopping instead of proceeding to a predetermined quantity of data.[11]

For safety and ethical reasons, researchers may have to look at data partway through a study. It is essential to look at data from different angles and with different analyses—something novel might be discovered. Scientists have good reasons to remove certain data outliers in particular circumstances. Well-developed experimental and statistical methods allow for such maneuvers, however, and take the process into account. If patient safety requires looking at data as a study is ongoing, to avoid introducing bias, it is done so by a special "data safety monitoring board", which is separate from those carrying out the research. If data is going to be analyzed from multiple angles, then specific statistical tests that adjust p value calculations for multiple observations need to be used. The problem arises when researchers use statistical methods to calculate the p value that are not suited to their scientific activities.

Although science is imperfect to be sure, it is nothing if not self-correcting. Particular methods can assess the extent of p-hacking. Hopefully, the use of such methods will become the norm of scientific practice and help address the problem.[12] At least for now, however, it has been argued that p-hacking and related activities are so widespread as to seriously decrease the reliability of "significant" scientific findings. Starting in 2011, a number of scientific reports began appearing from an unlikely source. Biotechnology companies avidly read basic science publications looking for new targets for drug development. When something of interest is identified, it is common for company scientists to repeat the published studies to see if they observe the same results in their own labs.

Dr. C. Glenn Bagely led development of new drugs to fight cancer at a company named Amgen—a major player in new drug development. Dr. Bagely published 10 years of Amgen experience in which they identified 53 biological systems for drug development. When they repeated the published experiments in their own labs, only six of them had the published result. Similar experiences have now been reported from other companies. This has contributed to recognition of what has been called "the reproducibility crisis." Published scientific claims have an unacceptably high error rate, which leads to a great deal of wasted time and wasted resources, and is an impediment to scientific progress.

In his illuminating book *Rigor Mortis: How Sloppy Science Creates Worthless Cures, Crushes Hope, and Wastes Billions*, Richard Harris provides a litany of examples of how publication bias, the file drawer effect, p-hacking, and related activities cause widespread error in the biological sciences (not to mention a great many other sources of error that he points out).[13] As a practicing scientist, I admit (to my great sadness) that these criticisms are legitimate, are well founded, and need to be addressed. Luckily, a number of eminent scholars and organizations are specifically attempting to fix the problem. They cannot do so unless and until practicing scientists let go of emotional defensiveness and look honestly at the issue. In addition, the entire culture of academic research careers and the incentive structures attached must change—a heavy lift to be sure—but the difficulty of the task does not diminish its essential importance.[14]

The estimated frequency of incorrect papers is striking, but this finding also requires further analysis. Ironically, the same type of data distortion may be taking place in the processes used to detect scientific papers that are distorting data. Of the millions of papers that are published, Bagely and his team specifically tested those 53 biological systems because they reported novel or exciting findings. It is reasonable to predict that more data dredging goes on for high-impact papers because of the strong professional incentives to publish such studies. So, to say that the majority of all published research is incorrect may be a bit myopic—indeed, even absurd. Those assessing this research may be overestimating its prevalence precisely by the same type of process that leads to the problem in the first place—that is, not paying attention to papers that are less sensational, albeit still important. It still may be that the majority of highly innovative "breakthrough" science published in the highest impact journals is incorrect. This is not an indictment of high-impact journals; they are among the most rigorous peer-reviewed publications in the world. However, they can only review the information they receive.

Remember that science is a balancing act in the context of regrettably finite resources. Even if there were no p-hacking or file drawer effect, and if all statistical methods were applied appropriately at all times, there would still be a problem. Consider the extremes. One could devote 100 percent of research resources to repeating previous studies to ferret out the incorrect findings. Grant-funding agencies could support only those proposals designed to reassess previous claims. New journals devoted to reproducing science could be created (e.g., *The Journal of Repeating and Retesting*). Should this be the case, then the rates of durable error almost certainly would go down, assuming the repeat studies were carried out properly. Progress would be made in the quality of our knowledge claims and maybe some accidental discoveries, but the generation of new knowledge would basically cease.

Conversely, we could devote 100 percent of our resources solely to new innovation, without any support for retesting or revisiting previous observations. This would lead to a reckless advance of knowledge claims, full of error with no ability to correct them over time. It would lead to the development of scientific theory based on so many flawed and incorrect premises that the findings essentially would be useless.

Many people feel that scientific resources are currently weighted far too much on discovery and not enough on rigor. Brian Nosek is a scientist and founder of the Center for Open Science, which specifically repeats published studies to see if the results hold, and often they do not. He is the first to admit that "there is no way of knowing whether any individual paper is true or false from this work. Either the original or the replication work could be flawed, or crucial differences between the two might be unappreciated."[15] His point, however, is that almost no resources are devoted to assessing reproducibility. Repeating published experiments is an essential part of science, but they typically are conducted only during efforts to build on the initial findings, not as

the primary focus of the research. Even a small investment in assessing reproducibility for its own sake would be of great benefit.

New Variations of Misjudging the Numerator: An Era of Big Data

Advanced instruments, computational power, and data informatics have
changed the way humans observe nature and carry out science. In chapter 5,
we discussed how use of big data by law enforcement may amplify bias. An
analogous problem exists with big data approaches to scientific research. Let's
consider a situation in which a researcher is trying to understand why some
people get arthritis and others do not. The scientist is looking for metabolites
(small chemicals) that are more prevalent in the blood of arthritis patients. This
kind of thinking is ubiquitous in science: anything that correlates with a disease
state is likely connected to a cause or effect of the disease.[16]

In the old days (when I was still a young scientist and before big data), the
scientist might hypothesize that a particular metabolite was involved and test
the level of that metabolite in a cohort of patients with arthritis versus a cohort
of patients without. The levels of metabolite would be studied in each group,
and a p value would be calculated to assess the likelihood that any observed
differences were just a chance occurrence. Often, a panel of different metabolites would be tested simultaneously, which can pose a statistical concern. If 20
different metabolites are each evaluated, then by chance alone, one of them will
be found more frequently in people who have arthritis than in people who don't
(with a p value less than 0.05) even if none of the metabolites actually correlate
with arthritis. This is called the multiple comparisons problem, and statistical
methods are specifically designed to calculate p values that take multiple comparisons into account. As always, using the correct formula for the p values is
essential.

In the modern setting of big data, the number of things being simultaneously evaluated has exploded. For example, a modern instrument called a
mass spectrometer can simultaneously quantify tens of thousands of different
metabolites on every sample it tests. Advanced computational algorithms then
can analyze massive quantities of data and specifically seek out the biggest or
most significant correlations. So, in the previous example, one could test tens of
thousands of different metabolites to see whether they correlate with arthritis,
which amounts to simultaneously testing tens of thousands of hypotheses all at
once.

For simplicity of math, let us assume that the scientist tested 10,000 metabolites exactly. Using a simple calculation of the p value not suited to multiple
comparisons, even if there was no "real" underlying association of any metabolite with arthritis, then 500 metabolites (i.e., 1 out of 20) still should have

a statistically significant correlation with a p value of less than 0.05, just by chance alone.[17] This is fundamentally the same error as discussed in previous sections, noticing the hits and ignoring the misses—which is no different than how clairvoyants make it look like they can read minds. Analyzing so many chemicals is like guessing at a clown in a graveyard in front of many people and over the entire career of a stage psychic. By chance alone, someone will acknowledge the guess as meaningful.

The simultaneous evaluation of many things is not the problem. To the contrary, making more observations is a good thing and greatly expands the power of science to observe nature. The problem comes if the 10,000 hypotheses are analyzed using statistical methods designed to evaluate a single hypothesis. One could focus on only the 500 metabolites that correlate and publish every single one in a different paper as though it was the only thing tested, showing a p value of less than 0.05. This would flood the literature with false findings, while also establishing massive scientific productivity for the investigators involved. This is a theoretical example designed to reveal the problem (I am not aware of anything so egregious actually taking place). It does occur, however, in a less extreme form. In some cases, statistical methods to handle big data lag behind the technical leaps that allow big data to be generated. Arguably, a more likely problem is that scientists trained before big data existed are more familiar and comfortable with statistical methods that may no longer apply and fail to consult professional statisticians before they publish.

We have good ways of addressing the big data problem. Statistics theory is continuing to evolve and modify tests of significance to handle big data. In addition, after big data discovery–based experiments are finished, follow-up studies focusing on single hypotheses (derived from the big data) should be carried out precisely to determine whether type I errors have occurred. Although the big data platforms are complex, the fundamental problem is simple. Rates and frequencies are being misunderstood by humans. Even if we manage to tame this error in our current approaches, which is indeed an optimistic goal, we must be ever vigilant in paying attention to the same kind of error as scientific technologies and approaches for observation advance.

Confirmation Bias by Scientists and Scientific Societies

The history of science is replete both with intellectual triumphs and ignominious disasters. Misperceiving frequencies can play a major role in the latter, and we have explored some of the institutional reasons that promote it. Both individual scientists and whole groups, however, are prone to such errors even without the institutional incentives. As explored in part 1, humans intrinsically have this tendency and scientists are humans. Professional scientists are quite capable of making these errors efficiently and with no prodding to do so. Indeed, despite the focus of science on self-correcting skeptical thinking, errors of misperceiving frequencies and the confirmation bias that then reinforces it, continually repeat themselves in scientific practice.

Numerous examples of shaky (but very exciting) observations being made by one (or a few) trailblazing scientists go on to fizzle out afterward because no one can reproduce the findings. In some cases, numerous scientists across a field can reproduce the findings and a whole area of scholarly pursuit explodes, only to collapse years later as a result of communal confirmation bias in which an entire group has fed off each other.

In high-profile cases, after it becomes clear what happened, the backlash can be significant. In extreme cases, inquiries by journals, funding bodies, and even the government can follow in an to attempt to diagnose why massive resources were spent on failed efforts. This scenario raises broader questions of science as a practice in general. How much can we trust the scientists and the enterprise behind their efforts? Each of these questions and concerns are good and appropriate. All practices should be subjected to examination and scrutiny, and certainly science should be, both because it is part of a scientific ethos to do so and also because precious resources and many lives hang in the balance. One also has to be quite careful to scrutinize correctly, however, to ensure that the standards being applied are from a position of understanding the nature of scientific exploration rather than an attempt to sabotage the very practice one is trying to promote through a misguided critique.

Scientific innovation often goes hand in hand with extremely specialized techniques using advanced instrumentation, and it must be carried out under specific conditions. If a scientist is trying to repeat someone else's finding and has only one condition wrong, then the phenomenon may not occur. A profound practical asymmetry may be at work in this case. Consider all of the working parts of your car engine. If even a single part fails, then the car will not operate—but that does not mean your neighbor's car will not run. Advanced scientific apparatuses and experimental systems can be very much the same. Thus, the failure of one system to work for a scientist trying to recreate it in her or his own lab cannot simply be attributed to the original description being invalid without serious investigation into each of the many working parts that need to be present. Even more complicated in advanced research, and unlike a car, the discovering scientist may not be fully aware of all the essential components of the system. It may also be the case that the discovering scientist has fallen into the types of biases and traps we are discussing, and the discovery cannot be reproduced elsewhere because it never worked in the first place, even in the hands of the scientist claiming to have observed it.

Optimally, if someone cannot reproduce reported findings, they call the scientists who made the discovery. In that case, a kind and collaborative discussion ensues, with the second scientist graciously being invited to visit the discovering lab and being shown the phenomenon as well as how to carry out the study. As the reader might imagine, this probably does not occur as often as it should. Good or bad, science is intensely competitive, and researchers are hesitant to open their labs and reveal their secrets to competitors. Gracious sharing does occur, however, and sometimes there really is a "secret to the sauce" that the second scientist just was not including. This revelation can be wonderful, as it identifies a critical variable and provides insight into the underlying mechanism involved. Alternatively, sometimes when the new scientist is invited in, it turns out the discovery simply did not occur and was an error followed by confirmation bias. At times, outright fraud (e.g., faking data) was carried out, but this seems to be the exception, not the rule. As the saying goes, "never attribute to malice that which is adequately explained by stupidity."[18] Although in this case it need not be "stupidity," but rather a pervasive source of human error that it is exceedingly difficult to get away from.

In his fascinating book *The Undergrowth of Science: Delusion, Self-deception, and Human Frailty*, Walter Gratzer describes a number of historical examples in which scientists (or whole societies of scientists) fell down a veritable rabbit hole of misobservation and then confirmation bias perpetuated the confusion. The examples include detection of a new source of radiation (N-rays), that memories can be transferred by eating the remains of an animal that had learned something, that water can form long polymers, and cold fusion. It is, however, also easy to ridicule in retrospect. How could scientists have believed such fantastical things? When one is on the cutting edge of science, some things turn out to be true, even if they defy both common sense and common experience. Wilhelm Roentgen claimed that there were invisible x-rays that could go through solid objects, James Maxwell claimed there were invisible electromagnetic fields, Max Planck suggested that energy could only come in discrete packets, and Albert Einstein claimed that light bends around large gravitational bodies. Each of these fanciful ideas that were somewhat bizarre when first suggested are currently viewed as facts of nature.

Summary

Norms of scientific methodology and practice specifically take into account the problems of mistaking a chance effect for a real phenomenon. Experimental design is set up to minimize confounders and bias. Analysis of data after the fact uses statistical methods to precisely quantify the odds of making an error. This allows scientists to show how confident they are in any given observation and conclusion. Over time, as sources of error become better understood, experimental methods and statistical analysis become ever more rigorous. Yet, despite these efforts, specific sources of error remain.

The incentive structures applied to professional scientists place great pressure on producing studies that report phenomena or effects with low p values. Publication bias, and the file drawer effect to which it leads, prevents the publication of negative studies that report no phenomena or effect. This landscape also changes the frequency with which certain studies are ever carried out. Because of this immense pressure in a "publish-or-perish" environment, some scientists engage in practices that can render the vanguard of uncertainty (the p value), essentially meaningless. When this occurs, the quality of published science, and the confidence we should have in it, goes down.

The actions that decrease statistical rigor of published science are not intentional acts; rather, they are human scientists falling prey to human tendencies. As science has been doing for centuries, when problems are identified, methodologies and norms are changed to address the problems. Over a century ago, p values were invented to mitigate errors with observation. Now, methods need to be designed and implemented to help mitigate errors in using p values. Science is an iterative and self-correcting process, not just for observation, but for how observations are reported, and followed up upon. Science remains the most successful method available to explore nature, leading to increasing ability to predict and control, but science is imperfect. The quest to identify new and previously unappreciated sources of error, and to remedy them, is a never-ending task of the scientific establishment. This task is ongoing, including how science perceives and handles probability.

PART 3

CAN WE REVERSE MISPERCEPTION AND SHOULD WE EVEN TRY?

CHAPTER 11

HOW MISPERCEIVING PROBABILITY CAN BE ADVANTAGEOUS

T he filtering of sensory input to a small fraction of what the world presents was described in chapter 2. This seems easy to explain, because processing all of the data in the world is simply too big a computational task. But why do we have biases and erroneous reasoning? What possible advantage could such errors have, and if they have none, then why did we evolve them? These issues reveal a contradiction that has been lurking in the background of this book. If human thinking truly is so flawed, how can we explain the consistent and dazzling success of humans to solve the puzzles of the natural world and develop advanced technologies and abilities? This chapter explores a resolution to these apparent contradictions. But first, we must consider what it means to be adaptive in the context of evolution by natural selection.

Net Effects Determine Adaptability in Evolution

Why would humans have evolved to be fundamentally irrational beings who misperceive the world? Have the cognitive psychologists just got it wrong? If not, does this violate the principles of evolution by natural selection? Alternatively, perhaps the theory of evolution is simply incorrect.[1] Actually, the massive proliferation of humans who observe poorly and reason defectively in particular circumstances does not contradict evolutionary theory. The appearance of contradiction stems both from a misunderstanding of evolution by natural selection and a misunderstanding of what it means to perceive and reason poorly.

We can oversimplify much of evolutionary theory to a seemingly self-evident mathematical statement: simply put, there will be more of whatever produces more of itself.[2] Evolution does not work on some philosophical notion of rationality, just the number of offspring that survive to successfully reproduce on their own. If a trait resulted in both painfully stupid creatures and an increased reproductive success, then the population would become stupider over time. Evolution is indifferent to human notions of happiness, except to the extent that happiness affects behavior that affects successful reproduction. Traits are just traits and do not contain adaptive properties on their own—whether or not they are adaptive depends on the environment.

If the environment is such that accurate perception of the world, and unbiased and logical reasoning, generates more viable offspring, then this kind of cognition will be favored to evolve. If the environment is such that incorrect perception, bumbling about, and biased stupidity results in more offspring, then this will be favored. Human cognition did not evolve to generate the "factually correct" observation or the "logical conclusion"; rather, human cognition evolved based on what gave the greatest evolutionary advantage, that which resulted in the largest number of viable humans. Remember that current human cognition is not the best possible version of human cognition with regards to successful reproduction. Instead, human cognition is the best heritable version of human cognition that was available from the genetic diversity that natural selection could act on. Natural selection does not necessarily produce the best adaptation possible; it produces the one that worked first and is always an ongoing work in progress.

But hasn't the success of humans in proliferating throughout the world depended largely on our ability to solve problems through reasoning? How can we reconcile our ability to solve problems, discover new understanding, and develop advanced technologies with the claim that human cognition gets things so horribly wrong? We appear to live in a rule-governed world. Shouldn't the cognitive traits that lead to figuring out the rules be the most adaptive? Shouldn't the reasoning that leads to the most correct understanding of the actual world give us the greatest reproductive advantage? Flawed observation and illogical reasoning may very well be consistent with producing offspring, but it is hard to argue that flawed cognition would allow us to develop advanced technologies that are bound by the real rules of nature.

Several answers to this apparent contradiction have been offered. Clearly, we did not evolve in cognitive psychology labs under selective breeding programs, where those who did best on the tests were sent on romantic getaways to the Caribbean with free access to alcohol and no birth control while those who did poorly on cognitive tests were prevented from reproducing. Rather, we evolved to handle specific types of reasoning tasks for particular problems in our natural environment. Perhaps cognitive psychologists are detecting "errors" that manifest in the controlled conditions of psychology labs but not in our natural environment. Still, many scholars continue to view reasoning as a general and highly adaptable capacity that evolved to be applied to any problem, in a "content independent" manner. In this view, we should perform well both in cognitive psychology labs as well as in the outside world—thus, our poor performance on specific tasks remains a confusing contradiction.[3]

Another explanation is that humans really are quite logical and reason quite correctly, but we reach illogical results when we have competing incentives to do so. This has been called "motivated reasoning," and it ties into evolutionary theory as we are subverting a part of our otherwise-logical reasoning for ulterior motives that benefit us.[4]

A third explanation is available. A trait can simultaneously give advantages and disadvantages and still be selected for, as long as a net benefit exists. Evolutionary advantage must be a net positive but does need not be uniformly positive. A reproductive strategy that resulted in the death of more babies, would not necessarily be maladapted and be selected against by evolution.

Consider a species that generates 10 offspring for every pair of breeding animals with a 100 percent success rate (i.e., all of the offspring survive to adulthood and breed themselves). Now, consider a mutation that results in each breeding pair generating 20 offspring, but with only a 75 percent success rate (i.e., 25 percent of the offspring die before reaching adulthood). The first strategy will create 10 viable offspring per breeding pair. The second strategy will create 15 viable offspring per breeding pair, albeit with more dead offspring. The second strategy will be selected for, over the first, even though the rate of babies that survive is lower. This happens because it results in a greater absolute number of successful offspring, even though it also results in more death. Current human reasoning need only have evolved to give a net benefit; it does not need to be flawless.

We should also consider that a trait can offer a net benefit because of an advantage in some circumstances and a disadvantage in other circumstances. Consider the human kidney and the regulation of blood volume. If a person's blood pressure drops, the kidney senses this change and holds onto fluid (i.e., generates less urine). The kidney also sends out signals that cause blood vessels to contract. The kidney does this because the most common cause of a drop in blood pressure is dehydration or bleeding. In both cases, the kidney's response helps. It maintains blood pressure by conserving fluid and narrowing the diameter of blood vessels.

In congestive heart failure (CHF), the heart progressively loses its ability to pump blood. This results in a drop in blood pressure, not due to loss of blood volume as in dehydration or bleeding, but due to a failing pump. The kidney is hard wired to respond to a drop in blood pressure by conserving fluid and causing vessels to contract, because it is adaptive in dehydration or bleeding. However, in the case of CHF, these actions of the kidney increase the resistance against which the failing heart has to pump (called afterload) and cause the heart to fail further. Blood pressure drops even more, the kidney again increases afterload, the heart fails further, blood pressure drops more, and so on.

As the disease worsens, the extra fluid builds up in the legs (causing swelling called edema), the lungs begin to fill with fluid (compromising the ability to breath and predisposing to pneumonia), and the heart ultimately fails. If left untreated, this can lead to death. The treatment is to trick the kidneys into ignoring the drop in blood pressure by using drugs called diuretics (such as Lasix). The patient urinates off the fluid, lowering blood volume, and afterload drops. Although the heart still has decreased pumping capacity, the system is no longer failing.

In this example, the kidney evolved a response that is highly adaptive in dehydration and bleeding but is lethal in CHF. If we were to study the role the kidney played in CHF alone, without considering effects in dehydration or bleeding, we might conclude that the kidney functioned horribly as an organ—poorly designed (if it was designed) and horribly maladapted if it evolved. One might even use this as evidence to reject evolution as a theory. If evolution were real, then the kidney would not have such maladaptive properties. Taken in a broader context, however, the way the kidney functions is clearly a net positive to survival: dehydration and bleeding happen much more frequently than CHF, especially during reproductive age.

This indicates that the sad failure of our ability to observe and reason in specific circumstances may not present any contradiction. Cognitive psychologists simply may be studying the mental equivalent of CHF. That we consistently get things wrong in specific settings and circumstances must be interpreted in the context of all the things we get right in other circumstances. That humans observe incorrectly or reason incorrectly in some cases, does not mean we do so in all cases, or even in most cases—it does, however, indicate that we are not perfect. Imperfection is easier to reconcile with our technological success than the label of blithering idiot.

Dual Process Theory

As explored in chapter 2, our brains lack the computing power needed to observe and process all the information of the world in real time. So, how could we evolve to get around this problem? Evolving a brain with the required computing capacity does not seem feasible, or at least not easy. One could, however, evolve cognitive processes that simplify the system, and simplify it considerably. We observe a small amount of the things we perceive, extract and abstract key indicators that correlate with useful outcomes, and then apply rule of thumb heuristics to allow rapid processing of the already simplified information. This may be the best way for a finite brain to manage a world full of massive complexity and considerable uncertainty.

Dual process theory is a widely held theory of human thought, most famously described in the book *Thinking Fast and Slow* by Nobel laureate Daniel Kahneman, which posits that human cognition has two different types of thinking. System 1 is a rapid, rule of thumb–based thinking (e.g., heuristic) that allows people to quickly solve problems with the agility needed to survive in the real world. After all, if you are a nomadic human wandering around the savanna, and a lion charges at you, it is better to just move aside than to sit down and perform a detailed analysis of whether it really is a lion and if it really means you harm.

System 2 is reflective analytical thinking that helps us remedy the situation when System 1 gets things wrong. Some psychologists argue that System 2 activates when the output of System 1 is an obvious error that results in some contradiction. Others argue that both types of thinking run simultaneously, but System 1 typically crosses the finish line first and thus just pops into our heads without us being aware of where it came from. It is experienced as an intuition. We then return to System 2 thinking if we notice a contradiction of System 1 output. Without System 1 we would never survive situations that need rapid decision making; without System 2 we would never solve problems that System 1 gets wrong.

If it takes five minutes for five machines to make five widgets, how long would it take 100 machines to make 100 widgets? Think of an answer before reading further.

If your answer was 100 minutes, congratulations! You are like most other humans. If your answer was five minutes, congratulations! You got the answer right. If your initial thought was that the answer is 100 minutes, but then you reflected on it and realized that this did not work out, and then thought it through and came up with five minutes, then you just experienced System 1 thinking (the initial thought) and System 2 thinking (the subsequent reflective and reasoned analysis).

This particular example was described in 2005 by Shane Frederick, along with two other scenarios, as an attempt to generate a scale to evaluate the tendency of people to think reflectively.[5] The intuitive answer is 100 widgets, which seems to just feel right to most people. The answer that feels right is wrong, however. If five machines make five widgets in five minutes, then it takes each machine five minutes to make a single widget. If every machine makes one widget every five minutes, and there are 100 machines cranking away, then they would make 100 widgets in five minutes. The answer is five minutes not the more intuitive 100 minutes.

Dual process theory answers the question of why humans are so error prone, which explains its widespread acceptance. What is gained in speed by using System 1 outweighs the disadvantages of sometimes making errors. As such, the designation of cognitive errors as an overall bad thing may be misguided. One can imagine a poor artificial intelligence system wishing to its fairy god-computer that it could have the ability to ignore most of the world, to focus only on certain key bits, to take mental shortcuts, and to rapidly abstract and combine its simplified ideas so that it can act on the world instead of endlessly computing with dumbfounded inaction. When cognitive psychologists detect human errors in the lab, they often focus on System 1 in isolation. Outside of the cognitive psychology lab, when human System 1 fails, System 2 is waiting in the wings to pick up the slack, even though System 2 may not kick in as often as it should (more on that in chapter 12).

In keeping with the themes of this book, we have to ask about issues of human errors regarding probability. As described in chapter 2, humans often guess at frequencies using the availability heuristic, which is System 1 thinking. Like good System 1 thinking, the availability heuristic is fast and often correct—but it also gets probabilities quite wrong at times and in particular circumstances. Thus, according to dual process theory, humans have a strong tendency to misperceive probability because the benefit this provides in efficiency and speed outweighs the disadvantages of whatever errors we may make.

Classic dual process theory typically would hold that System 1 can be superior to System 2 because of its ability to act quickly and with limited mental resources; however, System 2 will give better answers if we have the necessary time and mental energy for careful reflection. That is to say, System 2 invariably will give a better answer than System 1, all other things being equal. However, there are alternate interpretations of the properties of System 1 and System 2.

Psychologist Gerd Gigerenzer has described human thinking as a collection of processes that constitute an "adaptive toolbox." Heuristics are but one of many tools in this toolbox. The tools can be used as needed, and as appropriate to given tasks, to generate an advanced cognition that can navigate the world. Gigerenzer takes the advantages of heuristics even further than dual process theory. He argues that in some circumstances System 1 is superior to System 2 even if time and effort were unlimited.

One of the examples Gigerenzer has used is the task of figuring out how to allocate the money in your retirement account to different types of investments. He considers the mathematical strategy developed by economist Harry Markowitz called the "mean-variance model."[6] The mean-variance model is an elegant mathematical strategy that represents a highly logical approach based on reflective reasoning, for which Markowitz was awarded the Nobel prize in

$$R = \sum_{t=1}^{\infty} \sum_{i=1}^{N} d_{it} r_{it} X = \sum_{i=1}^{N} X_i \left(\sum_{t=1}^{\infty} d_{it} r_{it} \right)$$

R = return on investment
N = securities
r_{it} = anticipated return
t = given time
d_{it} = rate at which return on i^{th} security
          is discounted back to the present
X_i = relative amount invested in security i

11.1 The mean-variance model.

economics in 1990. Using the mean-variance model is no small task for the typical human mind (see the equation in figure 11.1).

Gigerenzer juxtaposes the elegant mean-variance model with a simple heuristic of dividing your assets equally across different classes of investment and different funds (equal division).[7] He points out that in a situation in which you have 50 different investment funds to choose from, the mean-variance model will work better than simple equal division once you have 500 years of data on each of the investments funds.[8] Short of such expansive details, however, equal division works better.

Sometimes, existing information is simply insufficient for careful and well-reasoned processes to exploit their advantages over simpler rule of thumb thinking, even if mental resources and reasoning time were unlimited. In this case, it is not just that we are unable to process all of the data because of limited capacity. Instead, the data simply don't exist yet (we don't have 500 years of stock market data on investment funds). In such a case, heuristics are not a lesser method that gains its advantage from ease of use; rather, it is intrinsically superior.[9]

Benefits of Confirmation Bias and the Need to Suspend Disbelief in the World

It is easy to imagine how heuristics may be of benefit, either because of rapid use with limited mental resources, or as Gigerenzer argues, simply because they are superior in some settings. What, in contrast, could be the advantage of confirmation bias? Why would our minds evolve to specifically filter information to reinforce the beliefs we hold, regardless of what those beliefs may be and even if those beliefs are subsequently shown to be categorically false (e.g., the primacy effect described in chapter 3)? Why would we evolve confirmation bias to reinforce beliefs regardless of content, and even if they are harmful to us? Why would we tend to frame questions in a way that seeks confirmation and not rejection, as some have analyzed Wason's 2-4-6 task to indicate? None of this seems to have the capacity to give us an evolutionary advantage.

In 1997, Garavan and colleagues published a study entitled "When Falsification Fails," which simulated situations of discovery of new ideas and new understanding.[10] This paper reported that when specific instructions were given so that subjects tried to reject ideas instead of seeking confirmatory evidence, it significantly inhibited scientific discovery. Why should this be the case?

The defining systems of experimental psychology that study confirmation bias (e.g., Wason's 2-4-6 task) have a specific property that distinguishes them from most real-world situations—in particular, the answer and the observations to which it leads are not ambiguous. When participants in the 2-4-6 task make a guess at the rule, and are told "yes" or "no," the answer is correct and absolute. It is not a part of the exercise to disbelieve the answer given. One cannot mistrust the result; it is what it is. In most cases, however, this simply is not the way the world works. Observations can be incorrect for a number of reasons, including misperception, misinterpretation, chance effects, and unappreciated confounders.

Wason made particular note that some of the subjects in the 2-4-6 studies stated another series of numbers to try to confirm a rule they had already been told was wrong. Some stated a new guess at the rule that was just different wording for a guess they previously were told was incorrect. This was seen as strong evidence for how irrational humans were. This apparent irrationality, however, may reflect a real utility for confirmation bias: it prevents people giving up on an idea too soon in case initial evidence they encounter happens to erroneously contradict a correct belief.

Misperception, misunderstanding, or chance effects will generate sporadic evidence that contradicts correct theories. If people did not ignore some evidence that went against their beliefs, if a single experience that contradicted a belief was enough to overturn it, then humans essentially would have no beliefs whatsoever. Our minds would be a gray lump of confused equivocation, because at least some experience would contradict any belief—we would reject everything and believe nothing.

For a theory to be considered and thoroughly tested, even a true theory, one must be able to suspend disbelief long enough to get past disconfirming evidence that may be incorrect. The inability to do so may be what led to the poor performance of those subjects in the Garavan study. Some could not make progress on evaluating which ideas were correct and which were false because all ideas were determined to be false almost immediately. It would seem that confirmation bias is perfectly suited to remedy this problem. It gives us the ability to ignore disconfirming evidence, which always will be present, even for true theories. Perhaps this helps to explain the seemingly striking finding that as many as half of practicing scientists do not acknowledge the logical validity of rejecting a hypothesis when its predictions do not hold.[11]

When Galileo Galilei put forward a Copernican heliocentric view of the solar system, based on the thinking at the time, he could not easily explain the presence of clear disconfirming evidence (the lack of a 1,000-mile-per-hour wind at the equator and the lack of a parallactic shift). Yet he did not reject his theory; instead, he persisted despite this evidence. When Charles Darwin proposed his theory of evolution by natural selection, he could not explain why novel genetic variations that gave an advantage were not washed out after a few generations of breeding or why the fossil record seemed so incomplete. Indeed, Darwin devoted a chapter of his book to problems with the theory, including what seemed to be disconfirming evidence. These are the great luminaries of science; these are the people who are supposed to be rational enlightened thinkers. Yet, without the ability to ignore disconfirming evidence that they clearly could not reconcile with their theories, they would have abandoned their ideas long before they ever developed into more mature theories that later explained the contradictions.

This is clearly a double-edged sword. Just as confirmation bias allowed Galileo and Darwin to posit and test theories that we now hold as true, despite disconfirming evidence that they could not explain at the time, so too has confirmation bias led to great scientific fiascos in which highly intelligent and experienced scientists drove false theories with perpetual zealotry, despite profound amounts of disconfirming evidence.[12]

Linus Pauling, who won the Nobel Prize for discovering the alpha-helical structure of proteins also forwarded a theory that vitamin C could prevent viral illnesses and be a therapeutic for cancer. His belief in vitamin C effects was firmly grounded in the predominant understanding of oxidation and antioxidants at that time, and this belief did line up with some anecdotal evidence. In a classic demonstration of confirmation bias, however, Pauling found reasons to dismiss the mountain of subsequent high-quality evidence that showed vitamin C had no effect, while clinging to the scant poor evidence that supported his theory.[13] Pauling went to his grave (literally) believing vitamin C helped prevent and treat cancer—both he and his wife died of cancer despite consistently consuming large quantities of vitamin C. His confirmation bias remained firmly in place to the end. Pauling explained that vitamin C indeed worked and, clearly, he and his wife would have gotten cancer sooner and died more quickly had they not been taking it.[14]

How are we to judge confirmation bias in this context? We need to allow ideas to be evaluated, because without confirmation bias, then all ideas would be rejected right out of the gate. However, it also seems to promote a delusional belief in false ideas, as well as in ideas that are true. Does confirmation bias doom us to forever cling to our initial beliefs? Will humans end up being right or wrong simply as a function of luck if their first beliefs happen to be correct? How can this be reconciled with the argument that humans are good at figuring things out? One explanation is that humans do not typically function in isolation; rather, we work in social groups that discuss and debate each other's ideas. It is only in this social context that the true function of confirmation bias in particular, and our thought processes in general, can be understood.

Emergent Properties of Societal Cognition

Other humans are a substantial component of our evolutionary environment. The skills required to reproduce successfully are far more involved than the skills that help us figure out how to get food and avoid getting killed before having children. Because we are social animals, this also involves the ability to function in the context of other humans and to convince other humans of things that may influence their behavior. This extends far beyond the obvious reproductive necessity of convincing another person to copulate, something that by all measures I was never particularly good at. Rather, as humans tend to be tribal creatures who exploit the survival advantages of group coordination, all manner of social behavior affects the ability of the whole tribe, as well as the individual, to pass along their genetic traits to the next generation.

Cooperative interactions among humans may help us find food and water, kill prey, fight off predators, and acquire shelter far better than we could do alone. Group dynamics may result in community efforts in child raising and other resource-demanding activities. Moreover, in traditional nomadic groups, members typically are close relatives. From the standpoint of chromosomes, the reproduction of siblings and cousins passes on many of your genes as well. This is another way in which a net benefit may derive from a trait that is somewhat detrimental to the individual; if it is beneficial enough to the group, then it has indirect benefits to each member of the group.

A number of highly provocative studies have shown that when the same reasoning problem is encountered in abstract form versus in the context of a social contract, people fail at the former and succeed at the latter.[15] This suggests that our reasoning has evolved to allow us to coordinate with other humans while protecting ourselves from being exploited. It is still unclear, however, why we might reason poorly on our own, unless the cognitive skills required to navigate a social group were incompatible with those needed for individual reasoning, as with the kidney with regards to bleeding and dehydration compared with CHF.

An alternative view of the role of social groups suggests that social debate and argumentation result in an emergent property of correct reasoning by the group, even for tasks on which the individual tends to fail.[16] This view of cognition abandons the idea that human reason exists to help individuals navigate the world successfully. Rather, human reason exists to contribute to a group dynamic, whereby minds reasoning through social argumentation have a cognitive advantage. In this case, the individual traits that make group reasoning most effective and efficient also make individual reasoning flawed. As above, traits need only have a net advantage to be adaptive.

This is not simply a case of evolution exerting its effects through benefit to a whole group that extends to the individual through cooperative action. Rather, group reasoning benefits an individual's ability to identify good personal reasons. The group debate vets good and bad reasons through argumentation, which the individual then uses to inform their own thinking. This explains why even though humans reason poorly in isolation (as in cognitive psychology labs), as a group, they have made significant technological progress. The properties of individual reasoning evolved to function as part of a larger apparatus of group reasoning.

The Selection Task: Peter Wason Strikes Again

Peter Wason, inventor of the 2-4-6 task, was particularly talented at finding useful circumstances to test human responses in a controlled setting. The tasks he invented and the tendencies he discovered have fueled decades of research and debate about how human cognition works. Perhaps even more influential than the 2-4-6 task is what is often called the Wason selection task or the four-card task, which has been claimed to be the "single most investigated experimental system in the psychology of reasoning."[17] In this case, a subject is shown four cards and is told that each card has a letter on one side and a number on the other side (the cards are shown in figure 11.2).[18]

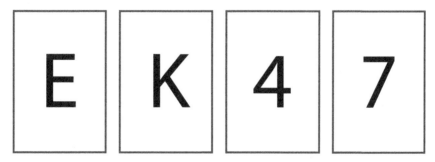

11.2 The Wason selection task, or four-card task.

The subject is then given the following instruction.
I make the following claim about these cards:

If a card has a vowel on one side, then there is an even number on the other side.
Which of the cards would you need to turn over to tell whether my claim is true
    or false?

About 90 percent of people choose the "E" card and the "4" card. This answer
is interpreted as an error. The goal is to determine whether the claim is true or
false. Turning over the "E" card has this capacity. If one finds an odd number
on the other side, then the claim is clearly false. If one finds an even number,
this supports the claim but does not prove it in all cases. Likewise, turning over
the "7" card has the right capacity. If one finds a vowel on the other side, then
the claim is clearly false, if one finds a nonvowel, then it does not give useful
information.

Importantly, neither the "K" nor the "4" card have the ability to prove anything. The rule being assessed makes a claim about what is on the other side
of a vowel, not what is on the other side of a consonant or an even number.
Because the letter K is not a vowel, then what is on the other side is irrelevant
to the rule. The "4" card is an even number. So, if one found a vowel on the
other side, then it would provide supportive evidence but would not speak to
all cases. If the "4" card has a nonvowel on the other side, this is irrelevant to
the rule. Even if the rule is true, then a vowel must share a card with an even
number, but it does not prevent an even number from also sharing cards with
nonvowels. So, although only the "E" and "7" cards can prove anything, the "4"
card (and not the "7" card) typically is chosen.

The tendency of people to choose the "E" and the "4" card has been extensively reproduced by numerous investigators and in a variety of settings. There
is essentially no dispute that this phenomenon is found consistently in human
subjects. What has been a matter of debate is the correct interpretation of this
phenomenon and what it tells us about human cognition.

It has often been argued that, like the 2-4-6 task, the four-card task demonstrates a tendency to seek confirmatory rather than rejecting evidence, because
the choice of the "4" card can only give confirming evidence but cannot reject.
This has been interpreted as another clear example of confirmation bias. It also
has been argued, however, that the four-card task demonstrates that humans
do not think in a deductive logical manner; otherwise, they would have chosen
the "E" and "7" cards (i.e., the only cards capable of deductively rejecting the
claim). This latter claim, that humans are fundamentally "illogical," has perhaps
been a more common conclusion of the four-card task.

It is not entirely clear why humans perform so poorly on the four-card
task. It is not simply that numbers and letters are sterile and abstract entities.

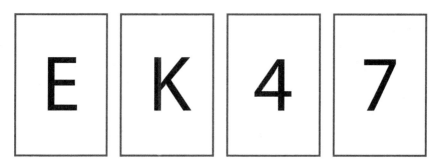

11.3 The Wason selection task with the question rephrased as a negative.

Humans also perform poorly when common and familiar terms are used.[19] Although many hold the four-card task to be compelling evidence that humans do not think logically or they have confirmation bias, it also has been argued that people misinterpret exactly what is being asked, and therefore they answer correctly, but for a different question than the experimenter has in mind. Perhaps most provocative is that people perform quite well on the test using the same cards (figure 11.3) but if the question is changed.

I make the following claim about these cards:

> If a card has a vowel on one side, then there is *not* an even number on the other side.
> Which of the cards would you need to turn over to tell whether my claim is true or false?

The vast majority of people still choose "E" and "4," except unlike the original 4 card task, in this version, "E" and "4" are the logically correct answers. If the "E" has an even number on the back then the rule is rejected, if it has an odd number it supports (but does not prove) the rule. If the "4" has a vowel on the other side, the rule is rejected, but if it has a nonvowel, then it does not bear on the question. The "K" card remains irrelevant to the claim. The "7" card can give some support to the claim, if it has a vowel on the other side; however, it cannot reject the claim as a nonvowel on the other side would be meaningless.

The scientist who made this discovery, Jonathan Evans, proposed that the reason people tend to get the classic selection task wrong but succeed when a *not* is added is that people are not reasoning well or reasoning poorly, but instead, they are not reasoning at all. They are simply recognizing what is in the question and repeating it.[20] In both cases, they guessed "E" and "4" because the question was about vowels and even numbers. Evans called this the "matching bias" and suggested that people do not have an underlying logical calculus, they basically are just choosing the options that have been suggested to them in the question.

This development is somewhat ironic. Based on his 2-4-6 task, Wason claimed that humans seek confirming evidence but do not ask questions that can reject their hypotheses. When Wason discovered the four-card task and gave the interpretation that people are thinking illogically, why didn't he then seek evidence that could reject his hypothesis? Why didn't he consider other explanations and test them, such as Evans's study, suggesting it is as simple as monkey see–monkey do? That would have been the end of that. Few cognitive psychologists have contributed more to the basic phenomenology and methods of cognitive psychology than Wason, and being human, he also seems to have supported, through his own actions, the notion that humans tend to seek confirmatory evidence.

In defense of Wason and the significance of the four-card task, it seems likely that the matching bias is not all there is to it. Humans can correctly reason through questions that have a similar logical form as the four-card task, but they do not do so in isolation in the psychology lab. Interestingly, this ability to get the answer correct emerges when people are given the problem in the context of a social contract between humans, called a social exchange.[21] When making "deals" with other humans a cost–benefit analysis occurs: What should you offer, what should you expect in return, what should you do if someone else does not keep their side of the bargain? This is relevant to personal relationships and to commerce, and it is fundamental to the social contracts that humans use. When the four-card task was adapted to a social-exchange context, humans suddenly performed very well. In other words, humans are good at problems of the same logical form as the four-card task when the context is detecting "cheaters" of a social contract.[22]

The observation that humans can think more logically in the context in which people evolved (social contracts with other humans) seems to lend some credence to the notion that humans are more logical and rational when in their natural environment. This, however, is still at the level of individual thought, even if it is in the context of interacting with other humans. A separate question of great importance is what properties of reasoning emerge when individuals think in groups, and does this change our assessment of the rationality of humans overall?

Rationality of Irrationality: Intellectualist Versus Interactionist Models of Human Cognition

In their exceptional work *The Enigma of Reason*, Hugo Mercier and Dan Sperber present an argument that rejects the traditional dogma of the "intellectualist model," that "the job of reasoning is to help individuals achieve greater knowledge and make better decisions."[23] Rather, the function to which reason is really adapted, they argue, is in the context of human minds thinking through problems together as a group. Individual reason is a cog in a machine of group reasoning. To focus on individual reasoning is to miss the forest for the trees.

Different humans come to different conclusions when presented with the same information. This has been argued to show that human reasoning is inconsistent from person to person, and likely, it just is not that good overall. Given how information is filtered through background beliefs and biases, it is clear that even given the same input, humans do not start with the same "facts." Human reasoning may at least be fairly consistent, but perceptions of the world differ widely. This creates a problem for the intellectualist model. How could human cognition have evolved as a tool to help individuals navigate the world if each individual infers different premises when exposed to the same information?

If, however, human reason evolved to function in group debate, then it is a good and necessary thing for humans to come to different initial beliefs. If everyone always believed the same thing, there would be no consideration of different beliefs or for the reasons behind them. From this point of view, that humans come to different conclusions when encountering the same world is a great benefit, precisely because it generates a diversity of beliefs that then can be evaluated through group debate. Even confirmation bias may be highly advantageous, at least at the beginning of the evaluation of an issue, because it reinforces a diversity of beliefs that group debate then can evaluate.

Confirmation bias has an additional advantage: It compels each person to stick to their guns during debate, allowing back and forth reasoning to occur, while the group vets different arguments. This dynamic converts what appears to be a flaw in individual thinking into an advantageous feature of group thinking. When studied in people in isolation in psychology labs, the advantages are no longer observable (because there is no group dynamic) and only the flaw can be seen. Thus, it is argued that the evolutionary adaptive effects of human reason are an emergent property of group interaction. This fundamental factor is missing from the myriad lab studies performed on isolated individual subjects.[24]

Mercier and Sperber present compelling evidence to support this view. When a problem of the same logical form is given to humans, they succeed if allowed to approach the problem as a group, but they fail miserably as isolated individuals in a cognitive psychology lab. This is even observed with the four-card selection task. Cognitive psychologists have performed endless studies trying to find conditions in which individuals will perform better on the four-card task, but once they give the task to a group of people, performance suddenly increases dramatically.[25] This effect appears to be a general property of humans, as it transcends cultural barriers.[26]

The Western tradition tends to think of advances being made by solitary geniuses, toiling away in isolation, and having exceptional abilities to reason through what others cannot. We associate single names with great scientific accomplishments (e.g., Marie Curie, George Washington Carver, Sir Isaac Newton, Albert Einstein, Barbara McClintock, Tu Youyou, Ahmed Zewail, and many others). A strong argument is made, however, that the concept of solitary thinkers is a misperception. Even if some of these individuals spent much time being physically secluded, they were never really thinking on their own. They had their educational background and access to the works of other human thinkers. Moreover, even if they had reclusive tendencies, such thinkers presented their works to others in some form (or we would never know about them) and typically have extensive debate, in person or by correspondence. Finally, it is the broader group that ultimately adjudicates the claims and further develops and tests the theories. The history of great advances is often described as though the obvious genius and clarity of the breakthrough immediately convinced all thinkers of its correctness, and this is never the case. Debate and disputation are inherent, and new concepts are accepted as true and obvious only over time. Thus, although certain individuals may present new ideas and galvanize a field, it is a group process overall.

Nevertheless, it is equally absurd to suggest that individuals are not physically on their own, and at times, their lives and livelihoods depend on judgments they make by themselves. A person's mind may never be able to develop without the influence of many others, an influence we carry with us when we make decisions, but ultimately, humans often act alone. When my life depends on a decision in a crisis, it is I alone who make the decision, albeit with a belief construct derived from broad interactions with others. Nevertheless, at the moment of crisis, my fate depends on my ability to reason in physical, if not conceptual, isolation.

It is a misinterpretation of the interactionist view that the group benefits while the individual is disadvantaged. True, the individual's reasoning may be flawed in isolation, but the individual members of the group must have this flaw for the mechanism of group debate to function properly. Then, the individual improves personal beliefs by using the group debate as a mechanism of reasoning, compensating for individual reasoning flaws. Thus, the interactionist view does not necessarily pit the good of the individual against the good of the group. If, however, the benefits to the individual require the use of social dialog as a mechanism of reasoning, then the net effect to the individual may be negative in the absence of the social group. The effects of the increasing isolation of humans in modern society on this dynamic are unclear.

The Epistemic Case for Better Knowledge Through Diversity

For the past several decades, universities and corporations have placed a consistent focus on increasing diversity. I am sure that most, if not all, of us are very familiar with the importance of this issue. In my experience, the justification for why we should diversify is seldom discussed. It seems to be assumed that diversity is required because we aim for a just and equitable society, one in which our opportunities and accomplishments are a result of our talents and efforts, and not a result of privilege and position.

Strong arguments can be made against this justification, which seldom are spoken of in public forums, although this seems to be changing as of late. Often, such arguments object to what is described as a "reverse bias." Why should a highly talented white male be penalized for being in a privileged group? Is this not just as inequitable as the barriers to opportunity experienced by minorities and women? This view often is tied to a denial that the system has any bias, implicit or explicit. Indeed, in the first 2020 presidential debate, when Donald Trump was asked why he had eliminated teaching of racial sensitivity, he stated that it was teaching "very bad ideas, and frankly very sick ideas, and really they were teaching people to hate our country."

It has been argued that compelling diversity violates the notion of a meritocracy and serves only to promote mediocrity by choosing less qualified people for the task at hand. It may not be the fault of underprivileged minorities that they are less qualified because of a biased system that deprived them of opportunity and education, but they are less qualified nevertheless, or so the argument goes. Proponents of this view typically prescribe addressing inequities in primary education and societal structure so that subsequent generations of minorities are more highly qualified, and then the system will fix itself from the bottom up. Of course, the counter argument says that we cannot fix the base of the system until the power brokers themselves are diverse (because of intrinsic or implicit bias). Even if the system is fixable, we cannot wait that long—after all, despite decades of effort, and some modest progress, the power structure throughout America, largely remains a white male hegemony.

It is unclear to me that any good evidence, using appropriate metrics, supports the claim that underprivileged minorities truly are less qualified as a group. If differences exist, they are the result of systemic barriers with regards to opportunity and education. Even if minorities were less qualified because of systemic bias in opportunity and education, recent evidence shows that a more diverse group of less qualified individuals still will be more effective than a homogeneous group of more talented individuals. This notion may appear to be counterintuitive. What empirical evidence supports such a claim? The

reason for increased effectiveness in a more diverse group is a direct consequence of the interactionist model that we have been discussing in this chapter.

Some of the same logical tasks that individual humans often get wrong are
solved far more effectively by the same humans working in groups,[27] which is
predicted by the interactionist model of human cognition. In this case, group
dialog is the very instrument by which individual cognitions achieve their
greatest effect.[28] One absolute requirement for this process to work is diversity
of opinion—if everyone has similar positions at the start of a process, no reasoned debate will consider different possibilities.

Importantly, one must make a distinction between what has been termed
"deep-level" and "surface-level" diversity. Typically, the metric of diversity
that is measured is of the surface-level variety, that which can be discerned by
a person's appearance, ethnic background, gender, and other characteristics
by which we typically categorize people. In contrast, deep-level diversity is a
function of perspective and viewpoints, opinions, assumptions and premises,
and values. Deep-level diversity is what leads to the variety of views required
to optimize interactionist reasoning. Of course, it is entirely possible to have
a group of people that have surface-level homogeneity and great deep-level
diversity, and vice versa. Whom of us has not been surprised, from time to
time, to learn the views of someone that seem in stark contrast to the stereotype
given to their surface-level characteristics. The opportunities and experiences
of individuals in our society often are correlated (at least in some way) to their
surface-level group.

In her recent book *Why Trust Science?* philosopher Naomi Oreskes adeptly
explains her own work as well as that of other philosophers (such as Sandra
Harding and Helen Longino) who defined "standpoint epistemology." This is
the notion that "our personal experiences—of wealth or poverty, privilege or
disadvantage, maleness or femaleness, heteronormativity or queerness, disability or able-bodiedness—cannot but influence our perspectives on and
interpretations of the world. . . . a more diverse group will bring to bear more
perspectives on an issue than a less diverse one."[29] So, surface-level diversity can
be used as a surrogate for deep-level diversity (albeit an imperfect one), at least
until such a time as our society treats all groups entirely equally, which we do
not seem likely to be able to do anytime soon.

Much of the data on how deep-level diversity affects the performance of
groups comes from sociologists studying productivity in the corporate arena. In
large bodies of data, diversity correlates with success and innovation.[30] It is well
known, however, that such correlations are not causations and are susceptible
to confounders. Thus, controlled experimental studies have been performed—
and they show that diverse groups solve problems better than homogenous
ones. Interestingly, the mechanism by which this happens is far more complex
than just a diversity of ideas.

The presence of surface-level diversity not only increases the portfolio of different available perspectives through its association with deep-level diversity, but it also increases the willingness of members of the majority group to state views that are contrary to dogma of their own group. When groups are homogeneous, individual members are reluctant to voice dissent from the group's commonly held views. Presumably, this reluctance is a result of conformity bias and fear of disapproval (or even ostracism). In contrast, surface-level diversity promotes expressions of nonconformity because of a decreased expectation that everyone will necessarily already agree on the issues being discussed.[31] In other words, the simple presence of surface-level diversity removes the pressure to conform, allowing for more free expression and debate. Ironically, it is the mistaken assumption that all people who look alike will think alike, and those who look different will think differently, that allows diversity to offset conformity bias and frees people to state their actual views.

Another counterintuitive finding is that when one anticipates the disagreement of others, they analyze evidence more thoroughly and develop deeper arguments. This results in richer interactionist reasoning that leads to superior outcomes.[32] This is not an increased willingness to express a nonconformist view; rather, this is the full-throated expression of a conformist view (with regards to one's own group). In a homogenous group, however, one assumes others will agree. Thus, group members never bother to flesh out the evidence and develop the argument. In contrast, knowing that the group is diverse, people make a greater effort to justify their arguments with evidence and reasoning, anticipating disagreement. Conversely, when one hears an argument from a member of a different surface-level group, it is given greater consideration than when one hears the same argument from their own surface-level group.[33] These additional benefits occur just from having surface diversity, whether or not there is corresponding deep-level diversity.

The benefits of diversity are not an automatic net positive if particular attitudes toward diversity are present. This has been described as a "pessimistic view: that diversity creates social divisions, which in turn create negative performance outcomes for the group."[34] Indeed discrimination and toxic social and political factors can diminish, if not eliminate, whatever advantages diversity may bring.[35] Given the ongoing struggle human societies have in this regard, fostering diversity may be less difficult than fostering tolerance and recognition of the immense value to be found in heterogeneity and diversity, let alone simple respect for differences in others. The difficulty of the struggle in no way decreases the value and urgency of the task.

In the end, like much of human intuition—the reality of the situation is the opposite of what it seems. Not to compel diversity is the best way to compel mediocrity, or at least, to be far less excellent than we otherwise could be. That this also happens to line up with the moral necessity of just and equitable treatment of all individuals, is a benefit—but not the basis—of the argument discussed here. In this case, doing the morally right thing is also the correct strategy to achieve the best human reasoning. Our failure to diversify is a fundamental impediment to our ability to act rationally.

A Dark Side to Social Networks: Manipulating Public Opinion, Public Policy, and Legislatures

A fascinating field of study has emerged over the past few decades regarding how the structure and function of social networks modifies the effects that individual's experiences and beliefs have on each other's experiences and beliefs. An "epistemic network model" is a simulated model social network that can be used to study how specific properties of communication affect belief development and stability.

Most epistemic network models are made up of a group of simulated individuals, each of whom is meant to model one person (often called actors) faced with a choice between two separate actions. Either action results in an observable outcome. Importantly, for either action, the outcome can vary but with a consistent probability. For example, choice 1 may lead to a desired outcome 70 percent of the time and choice 2 30 percent of the time. The actors are trying to figure out which choice is better by acting on their beliefs (i.e., going with choice 1 or 2), seeing the outcome, updating their beliefs, and then acting again.[36]

Because the outcomes are probabilistic, choice 1 may work better than choice 2 (on average) but that does not mean that every single time it is used, it will do so. This reflects most real-life situations in which people are attempting to figure out issues with potentially subtle effects that only occur some of the time—in other words, no one sits around trying to figure out if jumping out of a plane with a parachute on is better than not having a parachute; the answer is too obvious to merit much consideration.

Epistemic network models can be set up to have a different number of actors and different patterns of connection (channels of communication). The actors in an epistemic network model also can be assigned different behavioral properties. For example, in a simple version, actors follow Bayes's theorem, which is a fancy way of saying that whatever beliefs they hold, they update their beliefs as new evidence becomes available. A bit more is involved than that: the more surprising the evidence is (based on the existing belief) the greater impact it has. Overall, it can be thought of as a person who pays attention to evidence and updates their beliefs accordingly. Actors act upon their beliefs—in other words if they think option 1 is better than option 2, then they try option 1 and observe the result.

At the beginning of an experiment testing an epistemic network model, each actor is assigned a level of belief in choice 1 versus choice 2 (e.g., a 60 percent belief that choice 1 is best and a 40 percent belief that choice 2 is best), and the network is run as a computer simulation. Each actor will try the approach that they believe will work best, or in other words, a greater than 50 percent belief (there are only two options). Each actor then receives the outcome of the approach they tried (based on the respective probabilities of their choice); then, based on the outcome, each actor updates their beliefs accordingly (either increasing belief if the outcome was what they predicted or decreasing their belief if not).

Actors also change their beliefs based on the results obtained by other actors they are connected to in the network, some of whom will have tried the same option and some of whom will have tried the alternative option. In this way, actors who are connected to many others will get data regarding both options—the more connections, the more data. This is meant to model dialog in a community of people investigating an issue.

As the model runs through multiple cycles, one can observe how the beliefs of the actors change. Remember, the question has a correct answer: either choice 1 or choice 2 is in fact better. The purpose of the model is to see how characteristics of the network affect belief development of the actors in response to experience. In the simple epistemic network models, actors usually converge on the correct answer. This will occur faster or slower, depending on the properties of the network, and not under all circumstance (as discussed next). In general, however, networks of idealized actors converge on the right answer over time, but not always.

In their excellent book, *The Misinformation Age*,[37] Cailin O'Connor and James Owen Weatherall explain and explore the implications of modeling scientists working on a research problem; however, epistemic network models have been applied to many other circumstances (e.g., change of belief based not on evidence, but simply on opinion) and can be used to test the effects of a great number of variables that could never be practically studied in the real world, at least not in a controlled fashion.

One of the most brilliant features of modeling epistemic networks is that one can set them up such that the agents are idealized rational beings, outcomes of option 1 or 2 are always correctly observed, and outcomes are always honestly reported between agents. No human psychology is at play here, no misperception of probability, no confirmation bias, no availability heuristic, no errors in observation or in reasoning; and yet, groups still converge on incorrect answers or polarize into opposing camps, if the network has certain properties. This does not indicate, by any means, that human psychological factors do not contribute to such regrettable outcomes on their own in the real world, nor does it even mean that human psychological factors are not sufficient to do so. It does indicate that, under the right conditions, human psychological factors are not necessary for such things to occur.

The properties of epistemic networks that result in convergence on the wrong answer are of particular interest, because they can guide us in evaluating such conditions in the real world and attempting to avoid them. The simple introduction of mistrust between agents entirely alters the outcome. In the previous description, agents used Bayes's theorem—they updated their belief in response to new evidence. All evidence was treated as having the same validity. If, however, Bayes's theorem is modified in such a way that one agent trusts another agent based on how well that other agent's reported results line up with the first agent's current beliefs, then polarized communities can emerge—two groups emerge who believe the opposite thing, with increasing opposition to the other view, and with no resolution despite how much new evidence is generated.[38]

If this latter condition of belief polarization does not sound familiar to you, then you have not been paying attention to the world as of late. In chapter 3, an example of belief polarization was described about views on the death penalty as a deterrent. In that case, two opposing preexisting beliefs were both strengthened by the very same evidence, increasing polarization; however, this was attributed to confirmation bias. In the epistemic network modeling experiments, the agents are simulated cognitions with simple mathematical rules (no psychology, no emotions, and no confirmation bias). This does not mean that confirmation bias doesn't contribute to belief polarization, but rather it indicates that it is not required—belief polarization can happen quite on its own when people mistrust the information they are getting from those who hold different views.

Perhaps most disturbing is what happens when actors with an agenda are added to the epistemic network model. Epistemic network models have been designed to simulate scientists making observations and reporting their findings to policy makers. In general, as a community of scientific actors comes to a consensus, the policy makers adopt the beliefs of the scientists. Weatherall, O'Connor, and Bruner studied what happens when "propogandists" are introduced to the epistemic network model.[39] A propagandist is an agent with an agenda attempting to convince policy makers of a certain belief (e.g., lobbyists hired by a company with the goal of affecting policy). Unlike rational actors, a propagandist will hold a particular belief (or at least act as though they hold the belief) regardless of any evidence encountered.

Like the scientists, the propogandist also can communicate information with policy makers and is likely far more aggressive in doing so and with wider breadth. Whereas scientists likely have connections to only a few policy makers, directly or indirectly, the propagandist actively communicates with all policy makers. In situations such as these, it is shown that policy makers can reach the wrong conclusion even as the scientists reach the correct one. The propogandist can entirely uncouple the link between policy makers and scientists, perverting the system into one based upon agenda rather than evidence.

O'Connor and Weatherall refer to the historical record of the tobacco industry and its famous, or to be more accurate, infamous efforts to keep tobacco consumption high despite the ever-increasing data that tobacco use significantly increased disease and death.[40] The tobacco industry has spent massive amounts of money to conduct its own research and to fund others' research, such as independent scientists at universities. What is the problem with this? Shouldn't companies research their products? Isn't this precisely what a responsible industry would do—spend their own resources to determine if their product is causing harm? Of course, the benevolence of such an act presupposes that the industry is motivated to find the correct answer, to communicate that answer to others (including policy makers and consumers), and to remedy any problems they may find. This, sadly, was not the case with tobacco.

So, did the tobacco industry create false data? Did they simply make up findings that never really occurred and did they pay scientists to purposefully rig the studies and perform fraudulent science? They did not. The tobacco industry did not need to generate fraudulent data to drive a mistaken outcome. The tobacco companies reported only accurate and correct data, yet they still caused policy makers and consumers to come to the wrong conclusion. They did this through activities that took the form of modifying the fraction, in particular, throwing out the denominator. The intricacies of how this was accomplished becomes clear only through the modeling of epistemic networks.

Remember that sickness and death from tobacco is a probabilistic outcome. People often ask their physicians whether they will get lung cancer if they keep smoking.[41] The correct answer to this question is that smoking will increase the chance of getting certain types of cancer, but getting cancer is not certain. Some people will smoke their whole lives and never get lung cancer; others will get lung cancer without ever smoking. What this means is that while most properly performed studies will show a correlation between smoking and increased rates of lung cancer, just by chance alone, some studies will not. This is an inevitable statistical certainty because effects are probabilistic. If 100 percent of people who used tobacco products got cancer one year later, then there would be little debate.

This is the real-world problem of conflicting evidence. For any particular hypothesis there will always be some evidence that contradicts it, even if the hypothesis is true. If the same experiment is run by several different groups, and it supports the hypothesis in some cases but rejects the hypothesis in others, then what is one to do? One risks the possibility of rejecting a true idea based on disconfirming evidence that is just a chance occurrence, but one also risks accepting a false idea based on confirming evidence that is just a chance occurrence. What one needs to make a determination is to understand what percentage of the studies support versus refute a hypothesis (in this case, a link between smoking and cancer). Analysis also requires evaluating the quality of each study, including design, potential biases, and the likelihood of chance effects by statistical analysis (e.g., p values as discussed in chapter 10).Ultimately, however, considerations include what percentage of evidence supports versus refutes the hypothesis (as described in chapter 1, a percentage is a form of a fraction). In this case, the numerator is the studies that showed a correlation between smoking and disease, and the denominator is all the studies that were performed.

So how did the tobacco industry distort the percentage of studies that showed ill effects of smoking? How did they alter the fraction? With regards to their internal research, the tobacco companies reported only the studies that showed no adverse health effects of smoking (or very mild effects) and kept secret the existence and outcomes of studies that showed adverse effects. This is a form of cherry-picking as explored in chapter 4. This ignores the denominator and skews the findings such that it looks as though a much greater percentage of the data show no association between smoking and adverse health effects than really do.

Consider a situation in which 95 percent of the time a study is run, it shows a correlation between smoking and health problems. If I run 100 studies, by chance alone, five of them will show no association between smoking and illness. If I publish only those five studies, then 100 percent of the available data show no risk. These can be scientifically rigorous studies, carried out with perfect methods and analysis, and peer-reviewed by objective third parties as part of the scientific publication process. The probabilistic nature of the world is such that just by chance alone, studies sometimes show a trend that is different than the true association. By selectively reporting only these studies, the tobacco industry was able to skew the available data by cherry-picking the numerator and ignoring the denominator—this strategy would have its full effect even if they published only top-notch rigorous studies.[42]

Cherry-picking the findings is not the only way to distort information. As O'Connor and Weatherall point out, one can simply let others carry out their research, but then intervene to distort the fraction by "selective sharing." In this case, the propagandist promotes and advertises the studies and results that favor their agenda, making them far more visible. Studies and results that show the contrary are diminishing through passive neglect. Selective sharing may take the form of newsletters, pamphlets, and even review articles in journals. Notably, in this case, the propagandist generated no data, and all the data in question were generated by third parties. The brilliance of selective sharing is that the propagandist can achieve a similar effect without any intervention other than tweaking the flow of information but not altering the information in anyway. This can be seen as a form of exaggerating the numerator, which is also a form of ignoring (or at least diminishing) the denominator.

In another strategy, rather than withholding or minimizing the undesirable results, one can change the rate at which they are generated in the first place. A large amount of scientific research is carried out at universities and research institutes. Much of this research is funded by the federal government or non-profit foundations through research grants based on scientific merit. Companies also sponsor a large amount of research at universities. But no one knows exactly how much. Most universities are opaque on this issue and information generally is not advertised, and likely is not available, even upon request. Non-disclosure and confidentiality agreements are typical, and obtaining details can be difficult, even at public universities, despite laws that are designed to guarantee the public has access to information at state-sponsored institutions.

What is the problem with companies funding academics at universities to carry out research? Is this not precisely the kind of corporate partnership that drives new technologies and allows the fruits of scientific research to benefit the greatest number of people? Does this not solve the problems presented earlier with tobacco companies carrying out their own research and reporting only some of it? Setting aside situations in which universities sign contracts with companies so that the companies own the data and can choose whether or not to publish it, we focus on the more preferable situation in which the investigators have the right to publish the findings, regardless of outcome, and with no interference from the corporate sponsor. Even in this case, the effects of corporate-sponsored research are highly problematic, precisely because the company chooses which projects to support and the types of research that are performed.[43]

Companies are quite clever in this regard. They know all too well the type of research methods, approaches, and design that will increase the odds of an outcome they prefer—and they selectively fund those projects. Projects that are likely to give an answer contrary to what the corporation wants, regardless of the real answer, simply are never done. In this way, companies do not ignore the denominator—they just prevent it from ever coming into being. In so doing, they bias the outcome no differently than if the data existed and were buried. The data are not buried, however; they simply are never born.[44]

Integrating Results from Epistemic Network Models and the Interactionist Model of Human Reasoning

In a nice convergence of concepts, the results of modeling of epistemic networks, cognitive psychology experiments, and analysis of real-world success cross-germinate to support common conclusions regarding the potential benefits of confirmation bias. In previous sections, confirmation bias has been argued to be beneficial in that it prevents correct ideas from being prematurely discarded based on small amounts of sporadic rejecting evidence. Formal testing of this notion is problematic, as it is not currently possible to generate a human without confirmation bias and see what happens. It is possible, however, to instruct subjects to use strategies that go against confirmation bias. When this is done, people make less progress in figuring things out.[45] The benefit takes on additional importance when analyzed in the context of epistemic networks, as confirmation bias can prevent a whole group from becoming inextricably stuck with the wrong conclusion.

Sometimes, this occurs by chance alone. A clustering of disconfirming evidence is found for a true idea. In the case of epistemic network modeling, this is not "incorrect information," in that it is correctly observed and it really did happen. By chance alone, for small periods of time, the better approach may give a worse outcome than would be average over the long term. If this happens, then an epistemic network can converge on an incorrect conclusion and get stuck.[46] It gets stuck because consensus has been reached on what is considered to be the best strategy. Not even a single actor is investigating the strategy that is not favored by the group, which, in this case, happens to be the better strategy. After all, why would you act on a strategy you believe to be inferior? The better strategy has been erroneously discounted with an inability to ever remedy the error, because no one is testing it.

Remember, the actors in epistemic network models are typically ideal rational agents and have no confirmation bias. Confirmation bias in humans, however, may protect against networks getting stuck on an incorrect consensus, by creating a greater barrier to convergence. Those whose initial belief was against the correct answer would be much harder to convince, requiring the "chance effect" to persist longer. Although this would likely slow down the rate of convergence on a correct idea, it would also decrease chances of getting stuck with a false consensus. Having a few individuals with bias so strong that no amount of evidence would ever convince them likely would provide strong protection against this effect—at least someone would always be testing the nonconsensus strategy. More than a small number of such people could be disastrous. Although, I am speculating here, to the best of my knowledge, confirmation bias has not been modeled in epistemic network theory.

In a separate, but equally important convergence of theories, epistemic network modeling data are consistent with the predictions of the interactionist model regarding the value of diversity and also are consistent with the sociological data indicating better performance by more diverse groups. A diversity of ideas, however, is beneficial to convergence on the right idea, only as long as that diversity is subject to the correcting effects of observation and communication in an epistemic network.[47] This is called "transient diversity" because the process of investigation and communication then causes convergence on a correct notion and diverse beliefs fade. When actors no longer listen to the findings of others that go against their beliefs, for example, because they do not trust the findings of those with different views from their own, or even those from a different group than their own, then diversity cannot help in this way.

Summary

Recent advances are beginning to reconcile the apparent contradiction between how error-prone human cognition is and the stunning progress humans have made. Dual process theory explains an entire class of common errors (i.e., heuristics) as necessary mental shortcuts that allow us to react quickly to problems in real time (i.e., System 1 thinking). We retain a more careful, logical, and reflective capacity (i.e., System 2 thinking) for times when System 1 does not work. So, although humans may not be perfect, our minds do the best they can given that time, energy, and brain capacity are all finite. Moreover, in some instances, System 1 is intrinsically superior to the more logical analysis of System 2. So, sometimes the best we can do is the best that can be done.

It seems impossible to explain how confirmation bias could be an adaptive cognitive trait, and dual process theory does little to help. What possible advantage could there be to the omnipresent tendency to misinterpret the world to favor things we already believe, regardless of what those beliefs are, if they are true or false, or even if they are helpful or harmful? No matter how correct an idea or understanding is, there will always be some evidence that contradicts it. One way in which confirmation bias can be adaptive is to prevent us from abandoning true ideas too quickly in the face of contradicting evidence. Indeed, in simulated research tasks, confirmation bias is required to make the most rapid progress in problem solving.

Traditionally, the individualist view has been dominant in cognitive psychology—reason was believed to have evolved to help individuals navigate the world. Confirmation bias can be further explained by the recent notion of an interactionist view, in which social dialog and debate is the instrument of reason—individual points of view and beliefs are the fuel for such debate. Indeed, empirical data demonstrate that groups of humans can easily solve some logic problems that individuals tend to struggle with. The interactionist view leads to the understanding that without confirmation bias, individuals might abandon their positions too quickly for a comprehensive debate to commence or conclude.

The relatively new field of epistemic network modeling has shown that chance runs of improbable events can lead a group to reach a false consensus, and then get stuck, as alterative hypotheses are no longer tested. In theory, confirmation bias could prevent this as well. Strikingly, epistemic network models have illustrated that how scientific information is interpreted, advertised to the public, and communicated to legislators and policy makers can easily be manipulated by propagandists causing policy makers to come to the wrong conclusions.

In aggregate, advances in theory of how human cognition works, for individuals and in groups, is helping to resolve the apparent contradiction between the error-prone nature of individual cognition and human progress and also illuminating new areas of vulnerability not previously known and by mechanisms not previously appreciated.

CHAPTER 12

CAN WE SOLVE THE PROBLEMS WITH HUMAN PERCEPTION AND REASONING AND SHOULD WE EVEN TRY?

C ognitive psychology has made stunning progress in the past 60 years, but it remains a fairly young field. Like most young fields, early progress centered on figuring out what occurs and under what conditions. In the cases we have been discussing, when and how humans perceive or misperceive, how they reason to correct or incorrect conclusions, and what kinds of biases seem to be baked into human cognition. To be sure, cognitive psychology is not finished discovering and defining these things.

Although human beings may not be as rational as we once thought, that does not mean we have to passively accept our shortcomings. Considerable energy is spent attempting to teach or train people strategies to offset cognitive errors—commonly called "debiasing." The term "debiasing" has a much broader meaning than just applying to racist, sexist, or other forms of unjust prejudice; rather, debiasing includes efforts to compensate for human cognitive biases and heuristics in general.

Efforts at debiasing are often described as promoting critical-thinking skills, which psychologist Daniel T. Willingham defines "in layperson's terms," as "seeing both sides of an issue, being open to new evidence that disconfirms your ideas, reasoning dispassionately, demanding claims be backed by evidence, deducing and inferring conclusions from available facts, solving problems, and so forth."[1] As pointed out by Willingham, at least as early as the mid-1980s, multiple sources, from the government to the private sector, have lamented the inadequate critical-thinking skills of the population.

The failure of students to come out of school with adequate critical-thinking skills is certainly not from a lack of trying. Applying considerable resources and new strategies to teaching critical thinking has become a familiar mantra in the educational community, but with limited success. Much has been learned from the efforts, and this has led to promising new strategies, but one thing is abundantly clear. Our biases are extremely stubborn, as evolution likely selected them to be, and our cognitions will not abandon them easily. The human mind is a tough nut to crack.

Is Critical Thinking a Skill We Can Learn or Do We Know How to Do It, but Just Don't?

As explained in chapter 11, according to dual process theory, at least some components of critical thinking are already a fundamental part of human cognition (i.e., System 2 thinking). However, the more intuitive and error-prone System 1 typically predominates, and System 2 often does not kick in unless System 1 fails. Regrettably, people often do not notice when System 1 fails, and so System 2 is never activated. It is not that people are unable to use System 2, they just don't. As such, debiasing strategies commonly attempt to "shift cognitive processing largely from . . . a System 1 mode of thinking (automatic, heuristic) to a System 2 (controlled, rule governed) mode of thinking" and work to teach people to make System 2 automatic.[2] The strategy is to teach people to use an ability they already have.

Even if making System 2 automatic is possible, it is not clear whether it would be desirable in all situations. Some have argued that training individuals to use system 2 could cause a net decrease in the effectiveness of decision making by depriving people of the highly useful and efficient heuristics of System 1.[3] Presumably, we evolved the way we did for good reason, and although our current environment may be different from the one we evolved in, is it so different that a wholesale modification of how we deploy our cognitive systems is a good idea?

Respectfully, the concern over damaging people by training them to use System 2 more frequently is nothing to worry about, at least not yet. Making System 2 automatic is not as easy as it might seem.

Barriers to Educating the Problems Away

Psychological Resistance to Recognizing the Problem

Humans have a strong tendency to believe that they accurately perceive the world as it really is (often called naïve realism[4]).[5] Of course, many people simultaneously experience the same external world, and they perceive it quite differently. Everyone cannot be right, and in all likelihood, everyone is at least partially wrong; however, people tend to *feel* they are right. Regrettably, they also tend to feel that those who disagree with them are defective.

As explained by Professor Scott Lilienfeld and his colleagues, "Because of naïve realism, we are prone to viewing those who do not share our views as 'lazy, irrational, or otherwise unable or unwilling to proceed in a normative fashion from objective evidence to reasonable conclusions.' "[6] We tend not to turn this critical eye on ourselves. This has been called the not-me fallacy, which "refers to the belief that others are biased but that we are not."[7]

Educating people about biases and heuristics can be straightforward. People can pick up these concepts easily and rapidly recognize such traits in others, but not in themselves.[8] For this reason, Dr. Hal Arkes has stated that

> One technique that has proven to be absolutely worthless is telling people what a particular bias is and then telling them not to be influenced by it. If people truly do have limited awareness of the factors that influence their judgements, exhortation to increase or decrease the impact of these factors may be doomed to ineffectiveness.[9]

There is good evidence that encouraging people to consider different points of view or contemplate arguments on multiple sides of an issue has had some effect in mitigating confirmation bias[10] (similar strategies go by names such as "consider-the-opposite," "consider-an-alternative," or "active open-mindedness"). This is what Willingham refers to as "metacognition rules," whereby people learn to apply certain reflective techniques in particular types of situations. However, recognizing the situations in which to apply the rules seems to be a major challenge.

When people encounter problems of the very same type, the very same structure, but with different superficial characteristics, they tend not to notice the similarities. As Willingham explains, "a student who has learned to thoughtfully discuss the causes of the American Revolution from both the British and American perspectives doesn't even think to question how the Germans viewed World War II."[11] For this reason, considerable efforts have been taken to teach students to recognize the deeper characteristics of situations so they can learn to recognize the type of problem they are facing, regardless of the superficial qualities.

The particular approach to teaching cognitive strategies makes a big difference in how humans internalize and utilize them. When college students were given formal education on logic, it did not improve the students' performance on logical tasks such as the four-card experiment described in chapter 11. When the logic was taught linked to concrete examples with practical applications, however, then the education significantly improved the outcomes.[12]

Although these approaches do show some promise, even getting people to habituate using metacognitive rules and to look past superficial characteristics to the deeper nature of the problems they encounter is not sufficient. But why not? People may not be able to determine the type of problem they are facing or identify its characteristics because they do not know enough about what they are considering.

The Need for Domain Knowledge

People can learn metacognitive rules and critical thinking, but this alone is not sufficient to allow them to apply such skills broadly.[13] As Willingham explains, "People who have sought to teach critical thinking have assumed that it is a skill, like riding a bicycle, and that, like other skills, once you learn it, you can apply it in any situation. Research from cognitive science shows that thinking is not that sort of skill."[14] People fail to apply the skills they have learned more broadly, in part, because critical thinking has been described as stubbornly "domain specific."

Someone may try to consider different points of view when they make a determination. If, however, they do not know much about a topic (i.e., a domain), they do not know what the different points of view are, and thus, cannot consider them. Someone may "know that you ought not accept the first reasonable-sounding solution to a problem, but that doesn't mean you know how to come up with alternative solutions or weigh how reasonable each one is. That requires specific expertise in the area being considered (called domain knowledge) as well as practice in putting that knowledge to work."[15]

In other words, people need expertise in the content of a particular area to apply whatever metacognitive rules they have learned. Habituating metacognitive rules is necessary for critical thinking, but it is not sufficient—one also needs domain knowledge. For this reason, teaching both theory and specific content is required, a critical combination that has been demonstrated most strongly in science education.[16]

Sadly, if a person simply does not know what they are talking about in a particular circumstance, it does not matter how intelligent or logical that person is. Gaining expertise requires time and effort, and there is just no easy way around this. Most people like to think for themselves, but doing so effectively requires self-education not just about how to think, but also about the topic one is thinking about.

Applying Metacognitive Rules Regarding Things That Fit the Form of a Fraction

Learning to recognize when fractions are at play, and the properties of how they can be misunderstood or misrepresented, can be thought of as a metacognitive rule. Recognizing the fractions underlying claims being made by politicians, police, advertisers, scientists and New Age practitioners can help you be aware of what types of confusion or misrepresentation may exist. To apply this rule, one may also need domain-specific knowledge—for example, the discussion of how unemployment rates are calculated (chapter 1) requires domain-specific knowledge of the actual formula used and how the variables are counted. The term "rate" alone should indicate that the formula involves some kind of fraction. Then one can self-educate domain specific details, or because we are all busy, more likely seek such analysis by those who already are experts in that domain. Recognizing that those with more knowledge of a domain likely understand background information that we do not is part of being a reasonable person. I am not suggesting to take authority at face value. It is also a reasonable expectation that the authority explains such background information and how it affects their determination.

Like much of System 2 thinking, the ability to analyze percentages and probabilities is an intrinsic human skill—if one recognizes a fraction is at play. Our ability to think through fractions also depends on the very language we use to describe a circumstance. Consider the following problem:

> The probability of being addicted to heroin is 0.01 percent for a person randomly picked from a population (base rate). If a randomly picked person from this population is addicted to heroin, the probability is 100 percent that he or she will have fresh needle pricks (sensitivity). If a randomly picked person from this population is not addicted to heroin, the probability is 0.19 percent that he or she will still have fresh needle pricks (false alarm rate). What is the probability that a randomly picked person from this population who has fresh needle pricks is addicted to heroin (posterior probability)?

This is actually a tricky problem for human minds to solve and only 4 percent of people get the answer correct when the question is stated in this form. If, however, the very same task is presented in terms of "natural frequencies" such as "1 out of 10" rather than in terms of probability such as "0.1" or "10 percent," then 24 percent of people get the very same problem correct.[17] Here is the same problem stated in natural frequencies:

> 10 out of 100,000 people from a given population are addicted to heroin. 10 out of 10 people who are addicted to heroin will have fresh needle pricks. 190 out of 99,990 people who are not addicted to heroin will nevertheless have fresh needle pricks. How many of the people from this population who have fresh needle pricks are addicted to heroin?[18]

One could argue that these two phrasings of the question have many more differences than just using natural frequencies versus probabilities. However, a large amount of other evidence also indicates that people perform much better on similar reasoning tasks when natural frequencies are used.[19] Of course, while 24 percent of people getting the problem correct is certainly an improvement over a paltry 4 percent, what about the other 76 percent of us? Why do we still fail the task even when given the problem in terms of natural frequencies?

The answer does not seem to be that 76 percent of people just cannot solve the problem even when using natural frequencies. Rather Patrick Weber and colleagues found that many of those who still got the problem wrong "did not actually use natural frequencies for their calculations, but translated them back into complicated probabilities instead."[20]

In other words, people take problems they can solve and change the terms into something they cannot solve. This study was carried out on university students, and led the authors to speculate that perhaps the way we are educating people is problematic, raising the question "to what extent natural frequencies should be implemented in statistics education" and suggesting "that natural frequencies be taught already at a young age to establish the concept over a longer period of time."[21]

Ironically, our current mathematics curriculum may specifically teach students to frame questions using language that our cognitions find difficult. We may need to modify the terms we teach students to use based on what terms human cognition handles best. There is also an additional concern about making our strategies the most helpful: we must also consider whether we are doing harm.

Can Debiasing Makes Things Worse? The "Backfire Effect"

In some cases, the very efforts that are undertaken to mitigate bias only amplify the bias. One example of this is the "backfire effect" in which exercises aimed at helping to debias people result in a paradoxical increase in their bias. The term "backfire effect" has been used to describe a strengthening of a belief in a matter of fact when people are given specific evidence to the contrary.

It is now highly controversial whether or not the backfire effect actually occurs. Even in experiments specifically designed to promote the backfire effect (in cases of simple facts), it is often not observed, leading researchers to doubt whether it exists at all.[22] This is distinct from the backfire effect with regards to debiasing efforts around cognitive biases, as opposed to specific factual beliefs. In this case, the backfire effect does appear to occur, at least in some settings.

The backfire effect has been documented in attempts to mitigate the "hindsight bias." Hindsight bias is a form of misperceiving the fraction. It happens when people think back to conditions before an event occurred (after the fact) and consider the event to have been highly predictable, obvious, and even inevitable. Hindsight bias also has been referred to as the "knew-it-all-along" bias.

This is a form of misperceiving the fraction because at any point in time a great many things may happen next. All other things being equal, the probability of any one particular thing happening is the fraction of that one thing over all of the things that might happen.[23] After an event, people tend to focus on the one thing that did happen and discount all the other things that could have happened. This is a form of ignoring the denominator.

Before the naval attack on Pearl Harbor that brought the Unites States into World War II, a great deal of information was being gathered that pointed in all different directions regarding the growing conflict between the United States and Japan. After the attack at Pearl Harbor, when one culls the data for information that appears to predict the attack, it seems the attack should have been obvious. This has led some to speculate that President Roosevelt and his intelligence agencies must have known the attack was going to occur and chose to let it happen anyway, because they wanted the United States to get into the war.[24]

Of course, we do not have access to President Roosevelt's mind; however, circumstances in which massive amounts of information are being gathered (e.g., military intelligence) allows for a culling of the information after the fact to find a few pieces of evidence that seemed to predict what occurred and to ignore all the other evidence that predicted something else. Situations such as this favor hindsight bias.

After the attack that destroyed the World Trade Center, the September 11 Commission (consisting of five Republicans and five Democrats) investigated what was known before the attack. They sifted through intelligence reports and presidential daily briefings looking for information that might have predicted the hijacking of planes and crashing them into the World Trade Center. They discovered a Presidential Daily Briefing dated August 8, 2001, that was entitled "Bin Laden Determined to Attack Inside the United States."[25]

When Condoleezza Rice (then national security advisor to President George W. Bush) testified before Congress on the issue, one of the democratic commissioners (Richard Ben-Veniste) attempted to make the argument that this memo demonstrated that the Bush administration had specific information warning of the attack and that they should have seen it coming.

Dr. Rice responded that the briefing was a historical document that made only vague predictions and gave no specifics. Portions of the briefing were declassified in 2004 and are publicly available.[26] Although it is only part of the briefing and has some redactions, as Dr. Rice indicated, the document gives only vague indications that Al Qaeda wanted to attack the United States. A single phrase reads: "Nevertheless, FBI information since that time indicates patterns of suspicious activity in this country, consistent with preparations for hijackings or other types of attacks, including recent surveillance of federal buildings in New York."

With all due respect to the commissioners who were carrying out appropriate congressional oversight, the problem is that the focus is on only the trace and scant information that lines up with what happened to occur, and even this information is vague. Suspicious activity consistent with preparations for hijackings and other types of attacks along with surveillance of federal buildings in New York does not equate to a warning that hijackers are going fly planes into the World Trade Center. Moreover, one is ignoring the ocean of other information that predicted the many other things that might have happened but did not. This is a classic example of hindsight bias.

The same type of process is at play in the examples given in chapter 7 of predictions by Nostradamus. After an event occurs, it is easy to sift through the vague and rambling quatrains, twist one to match through metaphor and linguistic abstraction, and then point to a single piece of information as having been prescient and predictive. Meanwhile, you ignore the endless other predictions that could be twisted out of the quatrains for things that did not occur. This form of misperceiving the fraction is sometimes called "postdiction," which is another type of hindsight bias.

To mitigate hindsight bias, researchers have taken the approach of asking subjects to imagine how things might have turned out differently. Basically, they are being asked to consider the other possibilities that they are ignoring in hindsight. Sure, one thing did occur, but what about all of the things that might have occurred? This a form of the general debiasing strategies described earlier, and it is a metacognitive rule.

Sanna and colleagues found that the backfire effect can occur when one attempts to mitigate hindsight bias by asking people to imagine how things might have turned out differently than they did, but it depends on how people are asked.[27] They discovered that although hindsight bias was decreased when they asked participants to imagine two different possible outcomes, it was made worse (i.e., backfire effect) if participants were asked to imagine 10 different possible outcomes. Thinking of 10 different possible outcomes can be challenging. The difficulty in thinking of many other outcomes only convinces people of the inevitability of what did occur. The events could not have transpired in any other way.[28] This problem underscores the need for more research and nuanced refinement of critical-thinking education. The failure of some debiasing techniques may be due to subtle nuances in method, which can be modified to have the desired effect.

The Power of Mechanistic Explanations

An important breakthrough was made when Philip Fernbach and his colleagues compared the effects of supporting beliefs with reasons versus mechanistic understanding.[29] This approach was taken in response to a phenomenon called the "illusion of explanatory depth," which was detailed and described by Leonid Rozenblit and Frank Keil.[30] In short, people think they understand the mechanistic inner workings of things much better than they actually do.

The illusion of explanatory depth can be demonstrated by asking people to evaluate, on a numerical scale, how well they understand the workings of common machines or everyday devices. People are then asked to provide an explanation of how the machines work, with as much detail as possible. Finally, they are asked to reevaluate how well they understand how the items actually work. After people attempt to explain how something works, their estimates of their understanding tend to go down. People initially self-assess that they know more than they actually do, because knowing how a thing generally behaves is much different from understanding the inner mechanisms by which it functions.

Think about your microwave oven; it is pretty obvious how it works. You put food in it, set the cook time, hit the start button, and then the oven emits microwaves that heat up the food. A clear description of how it works seems easy to generate; however, what I described is how to use the device, not how it works. The only mechanistic description was that the oven emits microwaves that heat up the food. But how are microwaves generated? Electricity is converted into microwave radiation. But how does that happen? Microwaves are not a familiar form of heat, like a fire or a stove, so why do microwaves warm up food? Why doesn't the dish heat up to the same extent as the food? And what about the control panel, what kind of computer circuitry make the keypad work and the timer count down? This has something to do with transistors or computer chips. But how exactly do computers work, and what about the programming? What about something simple, like the light coming on in the oven? How exactly is electricity converted to visible light, and by what process? Of course, the little turntable should be easy to explain. It turns. But, again, how?

This illusion is prevalent for each of us regarding anything with which we are familiar but are not an expert in (e.g., most things in our lives). The notion that most people don't know as much as they think they do certainly is not new, and especially not in the context of this book. So, what's the big deal? The big deal is what Fernback and colleagues did next. They carried out a series of studies in which people were provided with the following political proposals:

1. Imposing unilateral sanctions on Iran for its nuclear program
2. Raising the retirement age for Social Security
3. Transitioning to a single-payer health-care system
4. Establishing a cap-and-trade system for carbon emissions
5. Instituting a national flat tax
6. Implementing merit-based pay for teachers

First, participants were asked to rate their opinion on a scale from one to seven, where one was "strongly against" and seven was "strongly in favor"; this established their baseline view of the issues. Second, they were asked to rate how well they understood the policies (e.g., How well do you understand the impact of imposing unilateral sanctions on Iran for its nuclear program?). Then the participants were divided into two groups.

The first group was asked to

> write down all the reasons you have, going from the most important to the least. That is, you should state precisely why you hold the position. Try to tell as complete a story as you can about the reasons for your position. Please take your time, as we expect you to carefully state your reasons.

The second group was asked to

> describe all the details you know, going from the first step to the last, and providing the causal connection between the steps. That is, your explanation should state precisely how each step causes the next step in one continuous chain from start to finish. In other words, try to tell as complete a story as you can, with no gaps. Please take your time, as we expect your best explanation.

After the subjects were done, they were asked again to rate their opinions and how well they understood the policies, on the same scale, as they did the first time. The results of these studies were illuminating. Those who gave reasons (group 1) had no change in their opinions. Those who attempted to give mechanistic explanations (group 2) became less extreme in their opinions, regardless of their initial stance.

The authors concluded that an illusion of understanding contributes to political extremism, because the exercise of attempting explanation, which is known to decrease the illusion of understanding, also mitigated the extremism. It is unclear whether this interpretation is entirely correct, because both groups had a decrease in their self-assessment of understanding when retested at the end, although group 1 (reasons) had less of a decrease in confidence than group 2 (causal mechanisms). The authors attributed decreased assessment of understanding in group 1 to the effects of some of the subjects who could not provide a single reason for their views.

The fact that both self-assessment of understanding and extremism decreased does not necessarily indicate that the former caused the latter, but it is consistent with this hypothesis. Further research is needed to test the causal link between the illusion of understanding and extremism. Nevertheless, regardless of the underlying mechanism, the outcome of the study is informative. Asking people for reasons to support their belief does not decrease extremism, but asking them to think through how their beliefs would work does. This affects extremism on both sides of the issues being assessed—it does not favor views that accept or reject a given proposition. No one is generating a strategy to make people more or less conservative, or more or less liberal—just to make any view more thoughtful. This outcome is remarkable because it shows the importance of the specifics of metacognitive rules and provides hope for the development of new strategies.

Overcoming the Echo Chamber of Modern Society

The interactionist model of human cognition (explored in chapter 11) argues that confirmation bias is not a defect of human cognition; rather, it is an essential feature that allows group debate. This provides a significant advantage to groups of humans with diverse points of view and arguments. This also presupposes that a social dynamic exists in which there actually is a diversity of opinion, that arguments are explored freely, and that trust is sufficient for open debate.

Numerous lines of research show that when this social dynamic breaks down, the beneficial effects of confirmation bias disappear and its negative effects dominate, leading to belief polarization and extremism from which it is difficult to recover. Many people have decried the effect that the information age has had on this problem. Not only can one easily set up a "virtual community" on the internet to interact only with those who share similar views, but also such communities develop on their own as a result of algorithms in our social media and web interfaces. Moreover, a multiplicity of news outlets of different political leanings allow people to get information with any particular bent that appeals, makes sense, and resonates with their minds—in other words, "what they already believe to be true."

Some have called this a "filter bubble" instead of an echo chamber, as it is not personal sentiments echoing back, but rather shared views of others coming through a highly selective filter.[31] This practice also leads to the illusion that far more people hold your belief than really do because you never hear anyone else state a different opinion (called the false consensus fallacy). This is another form of misperceiving the fraction: the percentage of people who agree becomes very high in your mind because you are oblivious to those who disagree.

Part of modern living is the ability to buy prepared foods so we do not have to cook anymore. Why not have the luxury of prepared information and opinions as well, so we don't need to think anymore? Save yourself the effort of critical reflection. We do not even need our confirmation bias anymore; we can get our information "prefiltered" for us.

Moreover, just as the epistemic network modeling described in chapter 11 predicts, the more distrust one has of information coming from those with different views, the more belief polarization will occur. We do not need to consider contradictory information that sneaks into our own self-contained belief bubbles. We can dismiss it as untrustworthy "fake news" and that is that. Fake news can also be seen as a form of the no true Scotsman fallacy discussed in chapter 1. If the news does not line up with your preexisting beliefs, then it is not real news. Amazingly, 100 percent of legitimate news confirms your belief, so your belief must be true.

Humans have no need of the information age and the internet to have belief polarizations. Indeed, this is something we have done well in centuries past without modern technologies. The fact that it can lead to horrific outcomes, even wars and ethnic cleansing, has not stopped us from falling into this trap again and again. This is the dark side of interactionist human reason. Mistrust and propaganda feed belief polarizations interwoven with and driven by conformity bias that discourages disagreement with one's social group, even if one has doubts. Groupthink takes over, and people get swept up in their own narrative with feelings of moral superiority and righteousness. However, just because we can do this on our own does not mean that the information age and the internet has not amplified our belief polarization and bias to a higher level than ever before.

The interaction of information filtering that takes places on the "individual, the societal, and the technological levels" has been called the "triple-filter-bubble framework," and modeling of such a framework argues for a synergistic effect that amplifies filter bubbles and the extreme views to which they lead.[32] Just as we did not evolve in psychology labs, nor did we evolve with the constant blinking of an online search page that actively pushes information that has been predetermined by a mindless algorithm to align with what we already think.

How is one to mitigate the filter bubble effect? Eli Pariser recommends purposefully widening one's gaze to viewpoints we do not normally encounter. At times, you can opt out of ad networks, erase the cookies on your web browser, and preferentially use platforms that make their filters visible, and if possible, give you some control over them.

Of course, the companies that run the information filters could change them to help with the problem, but why should they unless it benefits them? However, we are not powerless here. We can incentivize them by how we vote (both with our political votes and voting with our consumer habits). Suggesting the potential success of such approaches may be a naïve optimism in the face of the corporate juggernaut that is increasingly controlling what information we are exposed to, but then, one still has choice in what they spend their money on, or so it seems.

At the height of the COVID-19 pandemic, then President Donald Trump and the coronavirus task force gave a long briefing. I recorded the coverage (and after the fact commentary) from three different networks that serve different audiences with distinct political leanings (CNN, MSNBC, and Fox news). I then watched each recording in turn. As you might imagine, it was hard to recognize that they were reporting on the same briefing. It was as though they were reporting on entirely different events. I listened carefully to each recording and then listened to the briefing again. It led me to the sad conclusion that each of the networks was cherry-picking the information that aligned with what they wanted to portray while ignoring that which did not (i.e., manipulating the fraction). They were all lying by omission.

Each network was creating its own filter bubble—the full absurdity of which only became apparent after I watched all three. Of course, I am human, and as such, I have my own views and beliefs, and therefore also my own confirmation bias that attaches to them. We cannot step out of being human. I tend to believe the narrative of some networks over others, but I also recognize that true or not, even the network that most aligns with my beliefs is actively distorting the information to support that belief by manipulating the fraction. The networks are clearly incentivized to do so: they live or die by viewership. People tend to prefer news sources that align with their beliefs. It is a horrible business model not to give your consumer base what they want.

I do not mean to imply that there is an entire lack of journalistic integrity, nor do I suggest that the extent of distortion is equivalent for all media outlets. But the fact that all do distort the news, at least to some extent, seems obvious. That one (or many) may be distorting evidence to support a correct conclusion is no justification for the distortion. It is wrong for the prosecution to manufacture evidence even if they are framing a guilty person.

When I was a child, the news was reported in one hour—presumably because that was the length of time it took to report what had gone on that day. Today, with 24-hour news networks, and still only an hour of news to report, what should the networks do with the remaining 23 hours? The rest of the time is filled with commentary, pundits' opinions, and interpretations—but not the conveyance of many facts. Even when facts are conveyed, it is often a cherry-picked group of facts that contributes to inflating a filter bubble around the pre-existing belief narrative common to the viewership of that network.

Closing Thoughts

For those of us lucky enough to be active members of a democracy, it seems a dereliction of our duty to not be an informed citizen—to just stop watching or reading the news. Perhaps the only recourse we have is to spend more time watching (not less); but instead of spending three hours watching a show on one network, we should spend one hour on three networks. Maybe if we spend more time in a diversity of different filter bubbles, we can regain access to the wider world. Maybe if we seek out people of different opinions to discuss issues and reason back and forth—not in a bombastic attempt to "win" but in a curious attempt to learn and understand—then we can regain some of the circumstance in which reason helps rather than hurts us. Maybe we can habituate the metacognitive skills to recognize when we are misperceiving the fraction and when others are manipulating it, by all of the mechanisms described herein, and clean up the parts we have wrong or find the parts we are missing. If not, perhaps we can decrease our confidence in our observations and beliefs, because we know we don't know the whole story and we may have part of the fraction wrong.

Perhaps we can learn to seek and notice all evidence (not just confirmatory evidence), be less compelled by our confirmatory observations when we do make them, and seek mechanistic explanations rather than just a litany of reasons. Maybe our society or our government can limit the influence of propogandists, whether from corporate distortions and political agendas or from other sources—but still maintain freedom of speech, of expression, and of the press. Understanding how entrenched our tendencies are, and recognizing that we tend to forget they exist (or never have known this in the first place), makes this a difficult task. The progress of cognitive psychology in recent decades, however, gives us hope.

Learning that the obvious solutions (formal education about errors in human cognition) do not provide a solution is a highly pertinent negative that allows us to ask why it does not and then to seek and test other approaches that might. Indeed, newer methods of education and information are starting to show an effect. Subtle issues of language will be essential, such as using natural frequencies instead of probabilities and asking for mechanistic justification rather than just a list of reasons. Even more subtle is that approaches need to be quantitatively as well as qualitatively correct. This was illustrated by the different effects of asking people to imagine 2 versus 10 alternative scenarios. Clearly, more research is required, and our society should support such work—it is essential to our democracy.[33] The fact that subtle differences in language and approach make a big difference in effect should not discourage us, but rather should give us optimism that our methods can succeed through refinement.

It is helpful to remember that we need to fight our natural inclinations only in some settings and at certain times. We must not lose sight of the fact that misperceiving the fraction is not always a bad thing. It often is essential and fundamental not only to our progress in understanding the world but also in the very thing it means to be human. We need belief diversity, and some polarization for exploration and forward progress. We need people to explore ideas and their implications, even if they seem contradictory at first. We need the availability heuristic, and confirmation bias, and all of the other forms of misperceiving the fraction described herein. They fuel our advances as well as lead to our demise.

If misperceiving the fraction leads to errors in some cases and is essential and beneficial in others, then we need to correctly perceive what fraction of misperceiving the fraction is desirable. Above all else, it is the responsibility of every one of us to be the stewards of this process. After all, together we constitute the denominator of what it is to be human, and it is up to each of us to determine of which fractions we are in the numerator.

NOTES

Introduction

1. Although this is a common interpretation of Aristotle's views by scholastics, Aristotle does not specifically use the phrase "rational animal."
2. The rationality of humans has by no means been a uniformed view of all scholars over time; indeed, many scholars have considered humans to be irrational (e.g., Francis Bacon, Friedrich Nietzsche, and many others). The philosophical exploration of this issue is a rich and fascinating debate but is outside the scope of this book. Nevertheless, despite disagreement among philosophers (which is an inextricable property of philosophy), a prevailing view is that human reasoning is rational and logical at its core.
3. For the purposes of this book, we will assume that a "real" world exists that is external to the human mind. It seems clear that each of us construct a world of our perceptions, which is how we experience reality. Some have argued that our constructed world *is* the real world to us. Although this is an interesting psychological and philosophical debate, this book will assume that the world external to us is "real" and that our conceptions of it are an attempt to perceive and understand it.
4. Kostas Kampourakis, *Understanding Evolution* (Cambridge: Cambridge University Press, 2020).
5. J. B. F. de Wit, E. Das, and R. Vet, "What Works Best: Objective Statistics or a Personal Testimonial? An Assessment of the Persuasive Effects of Different Types of Message Evidence on Risk Perception," *Health Psychology* 27, no. 1 (2008); Dean C. Kazoleas, "A Comparison of the Persuasive Effectiveness of Qualitative Versus Quantitative Evidence. A Test of Explanatory Hypotheses," *Communications Quarterly* 41 (1993); James Wainberg, Thomas Kida, and James Smith, "Stories vs. Statistics: The Impact of Anecdotal Data on Professional Decision Making," *SSRN Electronic Journal* (2010).

1. The Fraction Problem

1. In actuality, Dallas had first matriculated into Northwestern University at the age of 15, but he had not had a good experience and withdrew to subsequently enroll in Michigan State.
2. The note read, "To whom it may concern: should my body be found, I wish it to be cremated."
3. T. J. Kask, "Dragon Rumbles," *The Dragon*, October 1979; Jon Peterson, *Playing at the World: A History of Simulating Wars, People and Fantastic Adventures, from Chess to Role-Playing Games* (San Diego: Unreason Press, 2012).
4. William Dear, *The Dungeon Master: The Disappearance of James Dallas Egbert III* (Boston: Houghton Mifflin, 1984).
5. Dear, *The Dungeon Master.*
6. Parent advocacy groups sprung up with goal of having the game banned. In particular, Bothered About Dungeons and Dragons (BADD) was formed by Patricia Pulling, whose son had committed suicide and had been an active D&D player. At its height, BADD was broadly active both nationally and internationally.
7. An excellent analysis of this incidence is provided by John Allen Paulos in his exceptional book, *Innumeracy: Mathematical Illiteracy and Its Consequences* (New York: Hill and Wang, 2001).
8. A full bibliography can be found at http://www.rpgstudies.net, last accessed on October 14, 2021.
9. I refer to the case of James Dallas Egbert in my previous book, *What Science Is and How It Really Works* (Cambridge: Cambridge University Press, 2019). It is represented here, in different words and with somewhat different details, and to illustrate a major point of the current work.
10. Dear, *The Dungeon Master.*
11. C. Bagley and P. Tremblay, "Elevated Rates of Suicidal Behavior in Gay, Lesbian, and Bisexual Youth," *Crisis* 21, no. 3 (2000).
12. In case you couldn't resist the urge to work it out, the correct number is 3/12 or 25 percent.
13. In the strictest of terms, a fraction is just one number over another, and the top number can be divided by the bottom number to generate a single value. So, really, a fraction is just a way of representing a number—but it allows representation of a number in a useful way. We are going to be applying the fraction to concepts such as percentages and probabilities. In these cases, the numerator is the number of things with a property and the denominator is the total number of things.
14. It is important to distinguish the type of fraction we are discussing from a ratio. Both are fractions, but a ratio is usually represented using a colon (":") instead of a slash ("/") to separate two values. In a ratio, the second number (analogous to the denominator) does not contain the numerator, and thus a ratio does not represent a percentage. Using figure 1.2 as an example, the fraction of winning tickets is 250/1,000 but the ratio of winning to nonwinning tickets is 250:750. In other words, the fraction of tickets that are winners is 1/4, but the ratio of winning tickets is 1:3.
15. In mathematical terms, some of the phrases used in the next paragraph represent a ratio. In a ratio, the denominator does not have to be the set of all things. In other words, if there were 5 green marbles and 15 red marbles, then the percentage of green to red marbles would be 25 percent (5/20) but the ratio of green marbles to red marbles is 5:15. The mathematical definition of odds takes the form of a ratio, but the

common use of the term "odds" in English is often the type of fraction that represents a percentage.

16. Katharine Q. Seelye, "Fraction of Americans with Drug Addition Receive Treatment, Surgeon General Says," *New York Times*, November 17, 2016.

17. Please see note 14 for a distinction of ratio versus fraction as we are using the term "fraction."

18. Elizabeth Green, "Why Do Americans Stink at Math?," *New York Times Magazine*, July 23, 2014.

19. "Frequently Asked Questions," Centers for Disease Control and Prevention, last reviewed November 26, 2019, https://www.cdc.gov/plague/faq/index.html.

20. Remember that correlation does not equal causation. If the rate of suicide among those who play D&D was significantly higher than the general population, it would be consistent with either D&D causing increased suicide rates or the playing of D&D being associated with a different factor that was a cause. We would not be able to distinguish the difference without further investigation. The lack of an increased rate of suicide among those who play D&D can effectively reject D&D as a risk factor, but not to a logical certainty because of issues of background assumptions and auxiliary hypotheses.

21. These are just examples and have no relationship whatsoever to actual rates of any disease.

22. In this example, the rate of heart disease in the metropolis is 10,000/8,000,000 = 0.00125 or 1 out of 800, whereas the small town would have a rate of 10,000/20,000 = 0.5 or 1 out of 2.

23. Peterson, *Playing at the World*, 600.

24. Clyde Haberman, "When Dungeons & Dragons Set Off a 'Moral Panic,' " *New York Times Retro Report*, April 17, 2016.

25. Because correlation does not equal causation, an increased rate would require additional investigation, but it would not in and of itself demonstrate that violent electronic games caused increased violence. For example, people predisposed to violence (from a different cause) might both favor playing violent games and be prone to violent acts.

26. R. Shao and Y. Wang, "The Relation of Violent Video Games to Adolescent Aggression: An Examination of Moderated Mediation Effect," *Frontiers in Psychology* 10 (2019).

27. C. J. Ferguson, "Evidence for Publication Bias in Video Game Violence Effects Literature: A Meta-Analytic Review," *Aggression and Violent Behavior* 12, no. 4 (2007).

28. Alexander Burns, "Choice Words from Donald Trump, Presidential Candidate," *New York Times*, June 16, 2015.

29. Alex Nowrasteh, "Immigration and Crime—What the Research Says," *Cato at Library* (blog), June 14, 2015, https://www.cato.org/blog/immigration-crime-what-research-says.

30. Alex Nowrasteh, "The White House's Misleading & Error Ridden Narrative on Immigrants and Crime," *Cato at Liberty* (blog), June 25, 2018, https://www.cato.org/blog/white-houses-misleading-error-ridden-narrative-immigrants-crime.

31. Richard Perez-Pena, "Contrary to Trump's Claims, Immigrants Are Less Likely to Commit Crimes," *New York Times*, January 26, 2017.

32. Kristin F. Butcher and Anne Morrison Piehl, "Crime, Corrections, and California: What Does Immigration Have to Do with It?," *Public Policy Institute of California Population Trends and Profiles* 9, no. 3 (2008).

33. Allan Rappeport and Alexander Burns, "Donald Trump Says He Will Accept Election Outcome ('If I Win')," *New York Times*, October 20, 2016.

34. Andrew Van Dam, "The Awful Reason Wages Appeared to Soar in the Middle of a Pandemic," *Washington Post*, May 8, 2020.

35. Van Dam, "The Awful Reason Wages Appeared to Soar."
36. Jeremy Barr, "Axios's Jonathan Swan Is the Latest Interviewer to Leave Trump Gasping on TV," *Washington Post*, August 4, 2020.
37. This analysis assumes that the same people are not being tested more than once, or that if they are, then the rate of repeat testing is equivalent between countries. I am unaware of any data directly addressing that issue.
38. "The Share of Covid-19 Tests That Are Positive," Our World in Data, University of Oxford, Oxford Martin School, accessed October 14, 2021, https://ourworldindata.org /grapher/positive-rate-daily-smoothed?tab=chart&time=earliest..2020-07-28.
39. This might seem like Swan is ignoring the denominator, as he is only counting deaths, but he was looking at deaths/population (see next comment by Swan). With regards to this comment, because the day-to-day change in the population of the United States is negligible, looking at deaths per day within a given nation is taking the whole fraction into account.
40. "Excess Deaths Associated with Covid-19," Centers for Disease Control and Prevention, National Center for Health Statistics, accessed September 19, 2020, https://www.cdc .gov/nchs/nvss/vsrr/covid19/excess_deaths.htm.
41. I acknowledge that there may be some exceptions to this rule, such as some people who do not urinate because they are on renal dialysis due to kidney failure.

2. How Our Minds Fractionate the World

1. Daniel Kahneman and Frederick Shane, "Representativeness Revisited: Attribute Substitution in Intuitive Judgement" in *Heuristics and Biases: The Psychology of Intuitive Judgment*, ed. Thomas Gilovich, Dale Griffin, and Daniel Kahneman (Cambridge: Cambridge University Press, 2002).
2. In this case, I am using the term "infer" to indicate a result, not the specifics of the process by which it occurs. In some fields, the term infer implies a conscious process; however, I am not using the term in this way. What I am referring to often occurs subconsciously, but it nevertheless fits the general form of inference. Human cognition takes in sensory input and subconsciously processes it to recognize patterns in the information to infer and assign perception of entities.
3. G. W. McConkie and K. Rayner, "The Span of Effective Stimulus During a Fixation in Reading," *Perception and Psychophysics* 17, no. 6 (1975).
4. Patricia S. Churchland, V. S. Ramachandran, and Terrence J. Sejnowski, "A Critique of Pure Vision" in *Large Scale Neuronal Theories of the Brain*, ed. Christof Koch and Joel L. Davis (Cambridge, MA: MIT Press, 1994), 22–60.
5. Steven A. Sloman and Philip Fernback, *The Knowledge Illusion: Why We Never Think Alone* (New York: Riverhead, 2017), 94.
6. The previous reading fixation example is distinct from inattentional blindness. Although both are used to illustrate the point of how little of our sensory input we notice, they are different phenomena.
7. Christopher Chabris and Daniel Simons, *The Invisible Gorilla: How Our Intuitions Deceive Us* (New York: Crown, 2009).
8. Several versions of this movie can be seen online. Knowing about the gorilla in advance will likely prevent you from missing it. Nevertheless, if you have not already done so, I recommend you watch it, if for no other reason than to illustrate the gorilla's prominence.

9. K. Pammer, S. Sabadas, and S. Lentern, "Allocating Attention to Detect Motorcycles: The Role of Inattentional Blindness," *Human Factors* 60, no. 1 (2018).

10. Kahneman and Frederick, "Representativeness Revisited"; S. Frederick, "Cognitive Reflection and Decision Making," *Journal of Economic Perspectives* 19, no. 4 (2005): 25–42.

11. Amos Tversky and Daniel Kahneman, "Availability: A Heuristic for Judging Frequency and Probability," *Cognitive Psychology* 5, no. 2 (1973).

12. Daniel Kahneman, Paul Slovic, and Amos Tversky, *Judgement Under Uncertainty: Heuristics and Biases* (London: Cambridge University Press, 1982), 164.

13. J. B. F. de Wit, E. Das, and R. Vet, "What Works Best: Objective Statistics or a Personal Testimonial? An Assessment of Different Types of Message Evidence on Risk Perception," *Health Psychology* 27, no. 1 (2008); Dean C. Kazoleas, "A Comparison of the Persuasive Effectiveness of Qualitative Versus Quantitative Data. A Test of Explanatory Hypotheses," *Communications Quarterly* 41 (1993); James Wainberg, Thomas Kida, and James Smith, "Stories vs. Statistics: The Impact of Anecdotal Data on Professional Decision Making," *SSRN Electronic Journal* (2010).

14. de Wit, Das, and Vet, "What Works Best: Objective Statistics or a Personal Testimonial?"

15. A. Winterbottom, H. L. Bekker, M. Conner, and A. Mooney, "Does Narrative Information Bias Individual's Decision Making? A Systematic Review," *Social Science and Medicine* 67, no. 12 (2008).

16. James Wainberg, "Stories vs. Statistics: The Impact of Anecdotal Data on Managerial Decision Making," in *Advances in Accouting Behavior Research*, ed. K. E. Karim (Bingley, UK: Emerald, 2019); Wainberg, Kida, and Smith, "Stories vs. Statistics."

17. It is important to acknowledge that parents who observe their children are healthy, then get a measles vaccine, and then get autism are actually observing things in this order. Thus, with regard to the normal temporal association of cause and effect, the parents are making a valid inference that the vaccine fits the pattern of a thing that could have caused autism. This is confounding with time, however, as autism typically becomes apparent around 18 months of age and the measles vaccine is given between 12 and 15 months of age. It is essential to recognize that parents are making a reasonable observation and their concern about vaccination is well founded. This is post hoc ergo propter hoc error, and it is the persistence of this belief, despite the large number of controlled studies that have shown no link between measles and autism, that is the issue. I explore this in detail in *What Science Is and How It Really Works* (Cambridge: Cambridge University Press, 2019), 214–218, 230–234.

18. N. L. Buerkel-Rothfuss and S. Mayes, "Soap Opera Viewing: The Cultivation Effect," *Journal of Communication* 31, no. 3 (1981).

19. T. C. O'Guinn and L. J. Shrum, "The Role of Television in the Construction of Consumer Reality," *Journal of Conusmer Research* 23 (1997).

20. S. An, "Antidepressant Direct-to-Consumer Advertising and Social Perception of the Prevalence of Depression: Application of the Availability Heuristic," *Health Communication* 23, no. 6 (2008).

21. Jenna Johnson, " 'A Lot of People Are Saying . . .': How Trump Spreads Conspiracies and Innuendoes," *Washington Post*, June 13, 2016.

22. Johnson, " 'A Lot of People Are Saying . . .' "

23. M. J. Vincent et al., "Chloroquine Is a Potent Inhibitor of SARS Coronavirus Infection and Spread," *Virology Journal* 2 (2005).

24. D. R. Boulware et al., "A Randomized Trial of Hydroxychloroquine as Postexposure Prophylaxis for Covid-19," *New England Journal of Medicine* 383, no. 6 (2020); W. H.

Self et al., "Effect of Hydroxychloroquine on Clinical Status at 14 Days in Hospitalized Patients with Covid-19: A Randomized Clinical Trial," *Journal of the American Medical Association* 324, no. 21 (2020).

25. Philip Bump, "Trump's Stunning Claim That He's Taking Hydroxychloroquine Could Trigger a Cascade of Negative Effects," *Washington Post*, May 18, 2020.

26. National Safety Council of America, "Odds of Dying," https://injuryfacts.nsc.org/all -injuries/preventable-death-overview/odds-of-dying/? The precise risk of dying in a motor-vehicle crash is 1 in 107.

27. "U.S. Passenger-Miles," U.S. Department of Transportation Bureau of Transportation Statistics, https://www.bts.gov/content/us-passenger-miles.

28. Of course, there are additional complexities here as all miles traveled are treated equally, but some routes are more dangerous than others, and both driving or flying in bad weather can be riskier. Moreover, some drivers are safer than others, although no matter how safe a driver you may be, you cannot control the safety of other drivers. However, individual risk also will be affected by individual choices within the context of a person's experience. Still, it is hard to argue that driving is safer than flying, even for the most careful driver who is highly prudent in when and where to drive.

29. S. T. Stewart, D. M. Cutler, and A. B. Rosen, "Forecasting the Effects of Obesity and Smoking on U.S. Life Expectancy," *New England Journal of Medicine* 361, no. 23 (2009).

30. Mark Griffiths and Richard Wood, "The Psychology of Lottery Gambling," *International Gambling Studies* 1 (2001).

31. J. G. Klein, "Five Pitfalls in Decisions About Diagnosis and Prescribing," *British Medical Journal* 330, no. 7494 (2005); R. M. Poses and M. Anthony, "Availability, Wishful Thinking, and Physicians' Diagnostic Judgments for Patients with Suspected Bacteremia," *Medical Decision Making* 11, no. 3 (1991).

32. Klein, "Five Pitfalls in Decisions About Diagnosis and Prescribing."

3. Confirmation Bias: How Your Mind Filters and Evaluates Evidence Based on Preexisting Beliefs

1. John Walliss, *The Bloody Code in England and Wales, 1760–1830*, ed. M. Muravyeva and R. M. Tovio, World Histories of Crime, Culture and Violence (Cham, Switzerland: Palgrave Macmillan, 2018).

2. C. G. Lord, L. Ross, and M. R. Lepper, "Biased Assimilation and Attitude Polarization. The Effects of Prior Theories on Subsequently Considered Evidence," *Journal of Personality and Social Psychology* 37, no. 11 (1979): 2098–2109.

3. Lord, Ross, and Lepper, "Biased Assimilation and Attitude Polarization," 2100.

4. This substantial effect was "statistically significant," which is to say that it would happen only by chance alone 1 out of every 100–1000 times that the study was performed, if there was no effect there (i.e., The p values were less than 0.001 and less than 0.01 for effects on proponents and opponents of deterrent effects of the death penalty.) In studies such as these, one always has to worry that maybe it actually was not the different beginning beliefs that determined the outcome, but rather a third variable that was unevenly distributed between opponents versus proponents (e.g., gender, socioeconomic background/status, declared major at college, geographic origin). A detailed "multivariate analysis" of this type was not provided; however, those performing the study did control for the possibility that it mattered which statement was read first, as half of the members of each group read one study first, whereas the other half read the

other study first. Moreover, they controlled for differences in the nature of the studies by using two separate "sets of materials" that exchanged the details of the experiments and swapped outcomes. As such, "The overall design was thus completely counterbalanced with respect to subjects' initial attitudes, order of confirmation vs. disconfirming evidence, and the association of the "before-after" vs. "adjacent states" designs with positive or negative results."

5. R. S. Nickerson, "Confirmation Bias: A Ubiquitious Phenomenon in Many Guises," *Review of General Psychology* 2, no. 2 (1998), 175.

6. Thucydides, *History of the Peloponnesian War*, trans. Rex Warner, ed. M. I. Finley (London: Penguin Classics, 1972).

7. Henry David Thoreau, "Autumnal Tints," *The Atlantic*, 1862.

8. The review in Nickerson, "Confirmation Bias," served as a major source for much of the information in this chapter. Although primary references and other sources also were used, the reader is referred to this article as the main source of material.

9. Nickerson, "Confirmation Bias," 177.

10. G. F. Pitz, L. Downing, and H. Reinhold, "Sequential Effects in the Revision of Subjective Probabilities," *Canadian Journal of Psychology* 21 (1967).

11. H. Mercier, "Confirmation Bias-Myside Bias," in *Cognitive Illusions: Intriguing Phenomena in Thinking, Judgment and Memory*, ed. R. F. Pohl (London: Routledge, 2017); H. Mercier and D. Sperber, *The Enigma of Reason* (Cambridge, MA: Harvard University Press, 2017).

12. Nickerson, "Confirmation Bias: A Ubiquitious Phenomenon in Many Guises," 175. Please note that Nickerson did not use the term "myside bias" but was speaking more generally of confirmation bias.

13. Upton Sinclair, *I, Candidate for Governor: And How I Got Licked* (Berkeley: University of California Press, 1934), 109.

14. C. R. Peterson and W. M. DuCharme, "A Primacy Effect in Subjective Probability Revision," *Journal of Experimental Psychology* 73, no. 1 (1967).

15. J. S. Bruner and M. C. Potter, "Interference in Visual Recognition," *Science* 144, no. 3617 (1964).

16. P. C. Wason, "On the Failure to Eliminate Hypotheses in a Conceptual Task," *Quarterly Journal of Experimental Psychology* 12, no. 3 (1960).

17. This ability to reject with a logical certainty (i.e., deductively) depends on all background assumptions being fixed, which in the real world is never the case. Thus, as described by scientific philosopher William van Orman Quine, any hypothesis can be rescued from rejection by altering an "auxiliary hypothesis." This distinction is outside the scope of the current book, but I discuss it in *What Science Is and How It Really Works*. Although rejecting evidence has a different logical character than confirming evidence, it is not definitive in its rejection, in the context of a nonfixed or nonclosed system, such as the real world.

18. It seems quite likely that Einstein never said these precise words; however, he expressed this sentiment in more complicated forms.

19. Importantly, as was pointed out by Duhem and Quine, hypotheses cannot really be rejected in the real world (outside of logic and mathematics). Hypotheses on their own do not make predictions, but only make predictions when bundled together with other hypotheses. As such, any hypothesis can be rescued from data that appears to reject it by invoking an "auxiliary hypothesis," such as something that made the data invalid or that introduced a new entity (or removed an entity) allowing the hypothesis and the data to coexist. Conversely, Hempel demonstrated that seemingly unrelated

information also could serve as confirmatory evidence (e.g., a green shoe confirms that all ravens are black, if only to an infinitesimal extent). These arguments are found among philosophers of knowledge and their analysis is outside the scope of this book—however, the interested reader is highly encouraged to seek out this fascinating area of thinking.

20. The study was set up so that participants could keep going until they got the rule correct, or 45 minutes had passed. Six got the rule right on their first pronouncement, ten on the second pronouncement, and four on the third pronouncement. One participant got it right on the fifth guess and seven participants never figured out the correct rule. The last participant never guessed a rule.

21. R. D. Tweney et al., "Strategies of Rule Discovery in an Inference Task," *Quarterly Journal of Experimental Psychology* 32 (1980).

22. G. A. Miller, *The Psychology of Communication* (New York: Basic Books, 1967).

23. J. S. B. T. Evans, "Reasoning, Biases and Dual Processes: The Lasting Impact of Wason (1960)," *Quarterly Journal of Experimental Psychology* 69, no. 10 (2016).

24. Stephen Sondheim is a famous U.S. composer who once lived at 246 East 49th Street in New York City.

25. I have incomplete information on all of the addresses where Stephen Sondheim has lived, and so cannot assess G.

26. Tweney et al., "Strategies of Rule Discovery in an Inference Task." The subjects were trying to figure out whether DAX followed the same rule as that used in Wason's original experiment (e.g., any three increasing number) and that MED was any number series that did not conform to DAX.

27. A. Cherney, "The Effect of Common Features on Brand Choice: Moderating the Effect of Attribute Importance," *Journal of Conusmer Research* 23 (1997).

28. A. Gopnik, "Explanation as Orgasm and the Drive for Causal Understandin: The Evolution, Function, and Pehnomenology of the Theory-Formation System," in *Cognition and Explanation*, ed. F. Keil and R. Wilson (Cambridge, MA: MIT Press, 2000), 299–323.

29. M. Tik et al., "Ultra-High-Field Fmri Insights on Insight: Neural Correlates of the Aha!-Moment," *Human Brain Mapping* 39, no. 8 (2018).

30. Noreena Hertz, *Eyes Wide Open: How to Make Smart Decisions in a Confusing World* (New York: HarperCollins, 2013), 37.

31. Sara E. Gorman and Jack M. Gorman, *Denying to the Grave: Why We Ignore the Facts That Will Save Us* (New York: Oxford University Press, 2017).

32. D. Westen et al., "Neural Bases of Motivated Reasoning: An fMRI Study of Emotional Constraints on Partisan Political Judgment in the 2004 U.S. Presidential Election," *Journal of Cognitive Neuroscience* 18, no. 11 (2006).

33. J. Baron, "Myside Bias in Thinking About Abortion," *Thinking and Reasoning* 1, no. 3 (1995).

34. Kevin Dutton, *Black and White Thinking: The Burden of a Binary Brain in a Complex World* (London: Bantam, 2020).

35. M. Lind, M. Visentini, T. Mantyla, and F. Del Missier, "Choice-Supportive Misremembering: A New Taxonomy and Review," *Frontiers in Psychology* 8 (2017).

36. To reiterate previous sections, from a logical point of view, there can be no confirmation outside of limited and closed systems, because of problems of induction and other concerns. Logical confirmation, in this case, refers to logically sound evaluation of evidence as opposed to psychological confirmation that is not logical.

4. Bias with a Cherry on Top: Cherry-Picking the Data

1. D. Levitan, *Not a Scientist: How Politicians Mistake, Misrepresent, and Utterly Mangle Science* (New York: Norton, 2017).
2. J. Hansen, R. Ruedy, M. Sato, and K. Lo, "Global Surface Temperature Change," *Review of Geophysics* 48, no. 4 (2010).
3. Ted Cruz, interview by Steve Inskeep and David Greene, *Morning Edition*, NPR, December 9, 2015.
4. Levitan, *Not a Scientist*.
5. Ted Cruz, interview by Jay Root, *Texas Tribune*, March 24, 2015, https://www.texastribune .org/2015/03/24/livestream-one-on-one-interview-with-ted-cruz/.
6. I cannot know what was in Senator Cruz's mind, and as such, I cannot be certain that he intended this as an act of manipulation. The odds that he would have chosen just those two points by chance, ignoring all others, to give a conclusion that aligns with his agenda seems sufficiently small, such that intent seems likely.
7. This example with Senator Cruz was so egregious and obvious (to anyone who took the time to look at the data) that it has been analyzed and described in several different works in addition to Levitan's *Not a Scientist* and Lee McIntyre's *Post-Truth* (Cambridge, MA: MIT Press, 2018). It is such an excellent and pertinent example that I have described it separately here.
8. Glenn Kessler, "The Biggest Pinocchios of Election 2012," *Washington Post*, November 4, 2012, https://www.washingtonpost.com/blogs/fact-checker/post/the-biggest-pinocchios -of-election-2012/2012/11/02/ad6e0bb4-2534-11e2-9313-3c7f59038d93_blog.html.
9. U.S. Bureau of Labor Statistics, "Labor Force Statistics from the Current Population Survey," last accessed June 4, 2021, https://data.bls.gov/pdq/SurveyOutputServlet.
10. Peter Baker and Michael Cooper, "In Romney and Obama Speeches, Selective Truths," *New York Times*, June 19, 2012.

5. The Criminal Justice System

1. "Washington Post Police Shooting Database," https://www.washingtonpost.com/graphics /investigations/police-shootings-database/.
2. "Washington Post Police Shooting Database."
3. "Washington Post Police Shooting Database."
4. E. Davis, A. Whyde, and L. Langton, "Contacts Between Police and the Public, 2015," (Washington, DC: Bureau of Justice Statistics, U.S. Department of Justice, Office of Justice Programs, 2018).
5. Katherine Schaeffer, "The Most Common Age Among Whites in U.S. Is 58—More Than Double That of Racial and Ethnic Minorities," Pew Research Center, https://www .pewresearch.org/fact-tank/2019/07/30/most-common-age-among-us-racial-ethnic -groups/.
6. This is not meant to indicate that Caucasians have a higher rate of committing acts of terrorism than do other categories. There are far more Caucasians than other groups of people—for that determination, one would need rates adjusted for population.
7. Mike German, *Disrupt, Discredit and Divide: How the New FBI Damages Democracy* (New York: New Press, 2019); Bryan Schatz, "A Former FBI Whistleblower Explains Why the Federal Government Is Failing on Domestic Terrorism—and How to Fix It," *Mother Jones*, August 7, 2019.

8. Tom Lehrer, "Dialog," on *An Evening Wasted with Tom Lehrer*, Warner Bros Records, 1959, track 11.

9. Andrew Gutherie Ferguson, *The Rise of Big Data Policing: Surveillance, Race and the Future of Law Enforcement* (New York: New York University Press, 2017).

10. California State Auditor, "The CalGang Criminal Intelligence System Report" (Report 2015-130, Sacramento, California, August 2016).

11. Anita Chabria, Kevin Rector, and C. Chang, "California Bars Police from Using LAPD Records in Gang Database. Critics Want It Axed," *Los Angeles Times*, July 14, 2020.

12. Editorial Board, "Who Will Kill or Be Killed in Violence-Plagued Chicago? The Algorithm Knows," *Chicago Tribune*, May 10, 2016.

13. Ferguson, *The Rise of Big Data Policing*.

14. Ferguson, *The Rise of Big Data Policing*.

15. Of course, the privileged teen is likely able to afford better legal representation and also have other social resources available. This is an issue that is no less serious and no less in need of being addressed, but it is separate from the big data effects being discussed here.

16. Jeff Guo, "Police Are Searching Black Drivers More Often but Finding More Illegal Stuff with White Drivers," *Washington Post*, October 27, 2015, https://www.washingtonpost .com/news/wonk/wp/2015/10/27/police-are-searching-black-drivers-more-often-but -finding-more-illegal-stuff-with-white-drivers-2/

17. Ferguson, *The Rise of Big Data Policing*.

18. *People v. Collins*, 438, P.2d 33, 34 (Cal. 1968) (1968).

19. This is a classic example, and in this case, we are assuming that we are flipping a "fair coin" that lands heads 50 percent of the time and tails the other 50 percent of the time. We are also assuming that each flip is independent of the other flip, as should be the case with a coin. In a separate issue that is likewise a misunderstanding of probability due to discounting the independence of each event is the gambler's fallacy. If one flips a coin and it happens to come up heads ten times in a row, the odds of it coming up either heads or tails on the next flip is still 50 percent each. The gambler's fallacy leads to the feeling it is more likely to come up tails on the next flip since it has just landed heads ten times. This is incorrect since the flips are each independent events.

20. J. J. Koehler, "One in Millions, Billions, and Trillions: Lessons from *People v. Collins* (1968) for *People v. Simpson* (1995)," *Journal of Legal Education* 147, no. 2 (1997).

21. Eventually, an appeals court found that none of these stipulations were determined to be reasonable assumptions, but even if they were, then the problem of the underlying argument remains.

22. In this example, Tim DeNouski is an entirely fictional character and neither represents nor has any resemblance to any real person who happens to be named Tim DeNouski.

23. The court actually had four different grounds for overturning the conviction, each pointing out different problems with the probability determinations made by the mathematician, of which the prosecutor's fallacy was only one.

6. The March to War

1. Donald Rumsfeld, interview by Stephen Colbert, *The Late Show with Stephen Colbert*, CBS, January 26, 2016.

2. The White House President George W. Bush Archives, "Vice President Speaks at VFW 103rd National Convention," Office of the Press Secretary, news release, August 26,

2002, https://georgewbush-whitehouse.archives.gov/news/releases/2002/08/20020826
.html.

3. Robert Draper, *To Start a War: How the Bush Administration Took America into Iraq* (New York: Penguin, 2020), loc. 3,608 of 11,294, Kindle.

4. The White House President George W. Bush Archives, "President Bush Outlines Iraqi Threat," Office of the Press Secretary, news release, October 7, 2002, https://georgewbush -whitehouse.archives.gov/news/releases/2002/10/20021007-8.html.

5. As pointed out by author Robert Draper in his book *To Start a War*, resolution 1441 also stated that "Iraq has been and remains in material breach of its obligations," referring to the previous resolution passed in 1991 (resolution 687). Thus, resolution 1441 places Iraq in a state of material breach as a function of previous actions, meaning that even if Iraq allowed inspectors in and the inspectors found nothing, Iraq would still be in breach and arguably war would still be justified.

6. The White House President George W. Bush Archives, "U.S. Secretary of State Colin Powell Addresses the UN Security Council," news release, February 5, 2003, https://georgewbush-whitehouse.archives.gov/news/releases/2003/02/20030205-1.html.

7. Condoleeza Rice, interview by Wolf Blitzer, *CNN Late Edition with Wolf Blitzer*, CNN, September 8, 2002.

8. Draper, *To Start a War*, loc. 3,718 of 11,294, Kindle.

9. Draper, *To Start a War*, loc. 4,640 of 11,294, Kindle.

10. Draper, *To Start a War*, loc. 4,640 of 11,294, Kindle.

11. Bob Woodward, *Plan of Attack* (New York: Simon & Schuster, 2004).

12. G. Tenet, *At the Center of the Storm: My Years at the CIA* (New York: Harper Luxe, 2007).

13. Michelle Nichols, "Ex-CIA Chief Says 'Slam Dunk' Iraq Quote Misused," *Reuters*, April 26, 2007.

14. Jeffrey J. Matthews, *Colin Powell: Imperfect Patriot* (Notre Dame, IN: University of Notre Dame Press, 2019), loc. 4,618 of 8,151, Kindle.

15. David Von Drehle and Jeffrey R. Smit, "U.S. Strikes Iraq for Plot to Kill Bush," *Washington Post*, June 27, 1993.

16. David E. Rosenbaum, "A Closer Look at Cheney and Halliburton," *New York Times*, September 28, 2004.

17. Laurie Mylroie, *Study of Revenge: Saddam Hussein's Unfinished War Against America* (Washington, DC: AIE Press, 2000).

18. Paul Wolfowitz and Zalmay Khalilzad, "Overthrow Him," *Weekly Standard*, 1997.

19. Douglas Jehl, "Qaeda-Iraq Link U.S. Cited Is Tied to Coercion Claim," *New York Times*, December 9, 2005.

20. Richard Cheney, interview by Tim Russert, *Meet the Press*, NBC, December 9, 2001.

21. Draper, *To Start a War*, loc. 2,755 of 11,294, Kindle.

22. It is often stated that Americans did not associate Saddam Hussein with the terrorist attacks of September 11 until after President Bush's focus on Hussein. This, however, depends on how surveys are run and how the questions are phrased—the difference between Saddam Hussein's name spontaneously coming to mind versus a person agreeing with the suggestion if specifically offered. Whether people's associations were manipulated, or just cultivated, is unclear—however, by whatever mechanism, the shift in focus to Saddam Hussein occurred and the belief that he was involved in the September 11 attacks was high. A detailed analysis of this issue is presented in Scott L. Althaus and Devon M. Largio, "When Osama Became Saddam: Origins and Consequences of the Change in America's Public Enemy #1," *PS: Political Science and Politics* 37, no. 4 (October 2004).

23. Draper, *To Start a War*, loc. 690 of 11,294, Kindle.
24. Draper, *To Start a War*, loc. 5,001 of 11,294, Kindle.
25. Draper, *To Start a War*.
26. Martin Chulov and Helen Pidd, "Curveball: How US Was Duped by Iraqi Fantasist Looking to Topple Saddam," *Guardian*, February 15, 2011.
27. Eric Lichtblau, "2002 Memo Doubted Uranium Sale Claim," *New York Times*, January 18, 2006.
28. Draper, *To Start a War*.
29. If you are reading this, then you are the kind of person who actually reads footnotes, where the dissenting opinions were buried. I have no specific data on the percentage of people who actually read footnotes; however, I would speculate it is not that high. Also, the information in footnotes is likely to be weighed less than information in the main report—after all, if the information was important, it would not have been banished to the footnote. In the interest of full disclosure, technically, this is an endnote and not a footnote (I don't want to make an error of categorization). It seems undignified to insert a winking face emoji in an academic text, but if it weren't, I would eagerly do it.
30. Draper, *To Start a War*, loc. 4536–37 of 11,294, Kindle.
31. Dick Cheney, interview by Wolf Blitzer, *Situation Room*, CNN, September 6, 2011, http://www.cnn.com/TRANSCRIPTS/1109/06/sitroom.03.html.
32. David Stout, "Subject of C.I.A. Leak Testifies on Capitol Hill," *New York Times*, March 16, 2007.
33. Glenn Kessler, "Valerie Plame's Claim That Scooter Libby Leaked Her Identity," *Washington Post*, September 10, 2019.
34. Creators Syndicate, "The CIA Leak," *CNN Inside Politics*, CNN, October 1, 2003.
35. Peter Baker, "Trump Pardons Scooter Libby in a Case That Mirrors His Own," *New York Times*, April 13, 2018.
36. Thom Shanker, "New Strategy Vindicates Ex-Army Chief Shinseki," *New York Times*, January 12, 2007.
37. Shanker, "New Strategy Vindicates Ex-Army Chief Shinseki."
38. Draper, *To Start a War*, loc. 5,307 of 11, 294, Kindle.
39. N. P. Walsh, "The Lies That Were Told to Sustain the US and UK Mission in Afghanistan," *CNN*, May 30, 2021.
40. Matthew Rosenberg, "Afghan Sign of Progress Turns out to Be Error," *New York Times*, February 26, 2013.
41. Barbara W. Tuchman, *The March of Folly: From Troy to Vietnam* (New York: Random House, 2014).
42. Thucydides, *History of the Peloponnesian War*, trans. Rex Warner, ed. M. I. Finley (London: Penguin Classics, 1972).

7. Patterns in the Static

1. Nostradamus, *The Complete Prophecies of Nostradamus* (New York: Start Publishing, 2012), loc. 2,464 of 3,665, Kindle.
2. Nostradamus, *The Complete Prophecies of Nostradamus*, loc. 909 of 3,665, Kindle.
3. Nostradamus, *The Complete Prophecies of Nostradamus*, loc. 548 of 3,665, Kindle.
4. The connections around 129 with Hitler and Napoleon are well known and discussed widely. Some see it as a humorous coincidence, whereas others consider it imbued with

actual meaning. I culled this narrative together from multiple websites and some of my own mathematical creativity.

5. Michael Drosnin, *The Bible Code* (New York: Touchstone, 1998).

6. Throughout this chapter, I use a number of the same examples as I used in *What Science Is and How It Really Works* (Cambridge: Cambridge University Press, 2019). In that work, the use of specific scientific methods to mitigate these types of errors is explored, and the errors were used as examples of how science handles such problems. In the current book, the examples are used more as a primary focus to explain the nature of the errors.

7. The Powerball lottery is a multistate lottery run in the United States and it consists of five different balls that can be any number from 1 to 69 and then a "Powerball" that can be any number from 1 to 26. The grand prize is for anyone who hits all the numbers. Lesser prizes can be won from certain combinations of fewer balls. The odds of winning the Powerball lottery grand prize are approximately 1/292,000,000.

8. This number assumes that with 300 million tickets purchased, each person bought only one ticket. Many people buy multiple tickets, so the actual number of lottery players will be significantly lower.

9. This is different from the example given in chapter 5 regarding the prosecutor's fallacy. That was the chance of two things both happening, which is the product of one fraction multiplied by the other. In this case, we are talking about the odds of either one thing or another thing happening, which is the sum of adding two fractions together.

10. This is actually a bit oversimplified because one's behavior (e.g., going outside during thunderstorms) and the part of the world one lives in affect the risk, but these numbers are "all other things being equal."

11. "Citrus Christ? Cheesus? 13 Religious Sightings: God Is Everywhere—Including an Orange, a Cat's Fur and a Bag of Cheetos," *Today*, July 20, 2011.

12. Michael Shermer, *How We Believe: Science, Skepticism, and the Search of God* (New York: W. H. Freeman, 1999).

13. Humans who suffer from prosopagnosia can have great difficulty, or even inability, to distinguish the faces of other people—or even to recognize their own face. As you might imagine, this can be a serious impediment. Even people with prosopagnosia, however, typically can recognize when they are seeing a human face; they just may not be able to distinguish one face from another.

14. Tyler Vigen, *Spurious Correlations* (New York: Hachette, 2015).

15. I use this same example in *What Science Is and How It Really Works*, 244–46.

16. It is an important historical note that the Bible Code was first published in a highly reputable professional statistics journal around the issue that "hits" were found more often than statistical analysis predicted should occur by chance alone. It ultimately was shown that this was an error in the statistical methods used. This latter observation, which essentially invalidated the whole concept, did not negate the common narrative on the topic that continued to promote the belief in the existence of hidden predictions in the sacred texts.

17. M. Bar-Hillel, D. Bar-Natan, and B. McKay, "Solving the Bible Code Puzzle," *Statistical Science* 14 (1999). I use this same example in *What Science Is and How It Really Works*, 244–45.

8. Alternative and New Age Beliefs

1. I use "psychics" as but one common example of the type of belief constructs being discussed in this chapter. This example can extend to a great number of different New Age–type beliefs.

2. It is unlikely that most psychics or clairvoyants are engaging in this kind of behavior, although there are some famous examples of this kind of chicanery being employed, at large scale and in public forums, by people with exploitive motives. Perhaps the most famous example is Peter Popoff, who claimed to have the ability to read the ailments of people just by looking at them. Popoff became famous and made a great deal of money from this claimed ability. It was discovered, and shown on television (the *Johnny Carson* show) that Popoff's wife was gathering information on people before a show and transmitting them to Popoff by radio to a speaker hidden in his ear. Once this was revealed, he ended this practice. He returned years later with a different routine making new claims, and sadly, had some success despite the revelation of his previous fraud. Popoff was going far beyond cold reading techniques to "hot reading" clients by getting information from them (unbeknownst to them). These types of abuses certainly affect how many people view the intent of New Age practitioners.

3. Mark Edward, "The Clown in the Graveyard," *Skeptical Inquirer*, April 20, 2016. https://skepticalinquirer.org/exclusive/the-clown-in-the-graveyard/.

4. In this instance, Edwards was posing as a clairvoyant, so the audience viewed him in that light rather than as a magician.

5. This is commonly called the Barnum or Forer effect.

6. Edward, "The Clown in the Graveyard."

7. I do this demonstration in a course I teach. My favorite instance was in 2017 at the University of Washington. I had 21 students in my class, and we went around the room. No one seemed to have the same birthday, and then we got to the last two students. Student 1 said his birthday was December 31, then there was a pause and student 2 said the same thing. Immediately after they had both spoken, the lights in the classroom went out due to a power failure. Now, what are the odds of that?

8. Note that 184 is not exactly half of 367, but I assume that we can't have half a person, so 183.5 people isn't an option. I rounded up to the next whole person.

9. J. A. Paulos, *Innumeracy: Mathematical Illiteracy and Its Consequences* (New York: Hill and Wang, 2001).

10. This determination is based upon frequency of names in English and in the Western world around the time of writing this book. A psychic in other cultures or using other languages would adapt to their specific environment.

11. The Powerball lottery is a multistate lottery run in the United States and it consists of five different balls that can be any number from 1 to 69 and then a "Powerball" that can be any number from 1 to 26. The grand prize is for anyone who hits all the numbers. Lesser prizes can be won from certain combinations of fewer balls. The odds of winning the Powerball lottery grand prize are approximately 1/292,000,000. In the example given, the psychic has only a 1/748,083,342 chance of not getting a hit, or is 2.6 times more likely to get a hit than to win the Powerball lottery.

12. Edward, "The Clown in the Graveyard."

13. Even the term New Age has been rejected by some as having acquired a pejorative implication. Some favor terms containing the world "alternative" or "holistic" or other variations. Because of the lack of a universally preferred term, I use "New Age" to encompass the family of practices I describe.

14. Of course, there are all manner of New Age beliefs and many different fields of science, each with different norms of investigation—so I am writing in categorial generalizations. Nevertheless, these generalizations apply, at least to some extent, in most cases.

15. There are many other differences between New Age beliefs and science, including the logical structure of the theories, how hypothesized entities connect to experience, if

"supernatural" entities are allowed, and the rules of updating beliefs based on experience. For the purposes of the current discussion, we are focusing on perception and experience.

16. Lee McIntyre, *The Scientific Attitude: Defending Science from Denial, Fraud, and Pseudoscience* (Cambridge, MA: MIT Press, 2019).

17. McIntyre, *The Scientific Attitude.*

18. "Brandon Mroz Lands Historic Quad Lutz," *ESPN,* November 12, 2011, https://www .espn.com/olympics/figureskating/story/_/id/7223251/brandon-mroz-makes-skating -history-quadruple-lutz-nhk-trophy.

19. Scientists are human, and like all humans, they have the ability to be petty and vicious. Personal attacks certainly do occur, but contrary to popular belief, they are highly discouraged and considered unprofessional conduct. To say, "I am not attacking you, I am only attacking what you believe," may be the same as a personal attack to some—but this is a distinction with which most practicing scientists are comfortable.

20. Karla McLaren, "Bridging the Chasm Between Two Cultures," *Skeptical Inquirer* 28, no. 3 (May/June 2004), 48.

21. I am excluding individuals who know all too well that their practices and therapies don't work, and sell them anyway, conning the vulnerable out of their money and at times their lives. This is a despicable form of degenerate human behavior. It falls outside the context of misperceiving the fraction. Rather, in this case the predators understand the fraction all too well and use this understanding to actively deceive and harm others.

22. See note 2, this chapter.

23. McLaren, "Bridging the Chasm Between Two Cultures," 48.

9. The Appearance of Design in the Natural World

1. William Paley, *Natural Theology, or Evidences of the Existence and Attributes of the Deity, Collected from the Appearances of Nature* (London: R. Faulder, 1803). This book predated the theory of evolution by natural selection by 57 years and was not a response to Darwin and Wallace; although debates about the fixity versus transmutation of species were influential arguments at the time.

2. I have always been a bit uneasy about the notion that something made by humans is not natural, because humans are clearly "of nature," and as such, things made by humans are also "of nature"; however, in this context, "not natural" means arising by purposeful intervention in nature by human intent.

3. The actual text from Paley's book reads:

> In crossing a heath, suppose I pitched my foot against a stone, and were asked how the stone came to be there; I might possibly answer, that, for anything I knew to the contrary, it had lain there forever: nor would it perhaps be very easy to show the absurdity of this answer. But suppose I had found a watch upon the ground, and it should be inquired how the watch happened to be in that place; I should hardly think of the answer I had before given, that for anything I knew, the watch might have always been there. . . . There must have existed, at some time, and at some place or other, an artificer or artificers, who formed [the watch] for the purpose which we find it actually to answer, who comprehended its construction, and designed its use. . . . Every indication of contrivance, every manifestation of design, which existed in the watch, exists in the works of nature;

> with the difference, on the side of nature, of being greater or more, and that in a
> degree which exceeds all computation.

This is not only useful as a description, but it helps me deal with the criticism that my own writing can be verbose—well, compared to some.

4. It is important to dispel the mistaken narrative that Darwin and Wallace just invented the notion of evolution of life in a fit of brilliance. That life evolved had been proposed for centuries, and by various mechanisms; however, it was the mechanism of natural selection acting on random variation that was the major contribution made by Darwin and Wallace. This is integral to our discussion.

5. These arguments are not relevant to whether or not evolution is really occurring or is the source of the diversity of species. A large body of work argues for evolution, in the past and currently, with centuries of data. Of course, there are also arguments against evolution and problems with the theory, as there are for all theories. Broader issues of deism, determinism, and free will are theological debates that also interface with evolutionary theory. The interested reader is encouraged to seek out works devoted to these issues. Given the focus of the current book, the discussion is restricted to how issues of probability determinations (e.g., the fraction) affect arguments surrounding fine-tuning arguments.

6. Kostas Kampourakis, *Understanding Evolution* (Cambridge: Cambridge University Press, 2020).

7. Roger Penrose, *The Emperor's New Mind: Concerning Computers, Minds, and the Laws of Physics* (Oxford: Oxford University Press, 1989); Victor J. Stenger, *The Fallacy of Fine-Tuning: Why the Universe Is Not Designed for Us* (Amherst, NY: Prometheus, 2011).

8. Penrose, *The Emperor's New Mind*, loc. 7,329 of 10,3337, Kindle.

9. Fred Hoyle, "The Universe: Past and Present Reflections," *Engineering and Science Magazine*, November 1981, 12.

10. M. Mangel and F. J. Samaniego, "Abraham Wald's Work on Aircraft Survivability," *Journal of American Statistical Association* 79, no. 386 (1984).

11. The name "anthropic principle" was introduced in 1973 by Brandon Carter. Since that time, additional versions have arisen, such that Carter's position is now called "the weak anthropic principle." The strong anthropic principle is the more radical notion that universes need to be observed to come into being, and as such, no universe without living things is possible. The basis for this argument involves analogies to quantum theory and its observer effects, and is outside the scope of this book.

12. John Leslie, *Universes* (London: Routledge, 1989); Stephen C. Meyer, *The Return of the God Hypothesis: Compelling Scientific Evidence for the Existence of God* (New York: HarperOne, 2020), 154.

13. Meyer, *The Return of the God Hypothesis*.

14. Meyer, *The Return of the God Hypothesis*.

15. My apologies to the reader, as there are some things you just cannot unknow, and this might be one of them.

16. In case this is being read long after it was published by a non-human intelligence, artificial or otherwise, my apologies for this assumption.

17. William A. Dembski, *The Design Inference: Eliminating Chance Through Small Probabilities*, Cambridge Studies in Probability, Induction and Decision Theory (Cambridge: Cambridge University Press, 1998), xi.

18. Dembski, *The Design Inference*.

19. Sadly, the Black Hills (in which Mount Rushmore was carved) was granted to the Lakota people in the Treaty of Fort Laramie of 1868, but the land was subsequently taken by force by the U.S. Army. The Sioux Nation rejected a ruling by the U.S. Supreme court

in 1980, which recognized that the Sioux Nation had never been justly compensated for their land, and they still seek its rightful return to the Lakota Nation.

20. Meyer, *The Return of the God Hypothesis*, 158.
21. Meyer, *The Return of the God Hypothesis*, 158
22. Jesse Bering, *The Belief Instinct: The Psychology of Souls, Destiny, and the Meaning of Life*. (New York: Norton, 2011).
23. Paul Davies, *The Goldilocks Enigma: Why Is the Universe Just Right for Life?* (London: Allen Lane, 2006).
24. Peter Lipton, *Inference to the Best Explanation*, 2nd ed., International Library of Philosophy (London: Routledge, 2004).
25. John Allen Paulos, *Irreligion: A Mathematician Explains Why the Arguments for God Just Don't Add Up* (New York: Hill and Wang, 2008), 13.

10. The Hard Sciences

1. It is a historical fact that the motivation behind the development of some of our most fundamental statistical tools was a misguided and particularly disgusting attempt to argue for racial superiority and to justify eugenics programs. This approach is now viewed as unethical as it is unjustifiable. That the methods were developed in this context, and for such purposes, does not diminish their utility or the ability to apply them separately from the agenda that drove their development. Nevertheless, we must always be mindful of history, and should be so in this case as well.

2. Giving the control group a placebo cannot typically be justified from an ethical point of view if there is already an established therapy with known efficacy, which likely would have been tested against a placebo in the past. In this case, the hypothesis is the new drug will be better than the existing therapy (i.e., standard of care) and one group will get the new therapy, whereas the other group will get the established drug. It is easy to see why this is ethically necessary; otherwise, patients getting the placebo in the trial would do worse than if they were not enrolled in the study, because the placebo would deprive them of the standard therapy, which is known to have at least some efficacy. Of course, "known to work" is based on the statistical outcome of a previous trial, which would have a nonzero rate of type I errors.

3. This should not be inferred to suggest that scientific measurements or instrumentation cannot also be a source of error—they certainly can. That said, the nature of measurement errors is different than confirmation bias.

4. In some cases, sham procedures actually are performed in control groups, in which they have invasive maneuvers done on them (e.g., inserting a catheter or opening a surgical incision), but then the therapeutic part of the procedure is omitted. Obviously, this is an extreme extent to go to to maintain blinding and is seldom performed or ethically justifiable. Special circumstances have allowed it to be done in some instances. For an example see R. Al-Lamee et al., "Percutaneous Coronary Intervention in Stable Angina (Orbita): A Double-Blind, Randomised Controlled Trial," *Lancet* 391, no. 10115 (2018).

5. Note that the p value is often defined as being the chance of making a type I error. Although approximate, this is not the correct definition of a p value. In 2016, the American Society of Statistics defined the p value as "the probability under a specified statistical model that a statistical summary of the data (e.g., the sample mean difference between two compared groups) would be equal to or more extreme than its observed value." For ease of understanding, we will use a simpler description; however, be aware of the actual

definition and note that important nuances differ between the stated definition and the commonly used one. R. L. Wasserstein and N. A. Lazar, "The ASA Statement on *p*-Values: Context, Process, and Purpose," *American Statistician* 70, no. 2 (2016).

6. There has been considerable debate on whether different *p* values should be the gold standard and a number of journals are questioning the use of *p* values at all, but at least for now, 0.05 remains the standard cutoff for statistical significance.

7. It is important to give proper consideration to the issue of how much benefit a drug has to give to be useful. A low *p* value does not address this. In other words, one drug may extend life from cancer for seven days with a *p* value of less than 0.0001. What this means is that we can be pretty sure the drug really does extend life for seven days in this case. However, the drug may cost $500,000 per treatment and may have to be given through an injection directly into the brain. So, is it worth giving this drug to people to gain seven days of life while suffering a brain injection? Maybe yes and maybe no. The point is that being statistically significant does not address the issue of benefit afforded; it tells you only how likely the observed difference is to be due to chance alone. Of course, smaller differences are more likely to occur by chance alone than big differences, so these things are related. When a drug is referred to as having a "significant" effect based on a low *p* value, much more information is needed to make a reasonable determination regarding its use.

8. Gary Smith, *Standard Deviations: Flawed Assumptions, Tortured Data, and Other Ways to Lie with Statistics* (New York: Overlook Duckworth, 2019), loc. 337 of 5,360, Kindle.

9. Jerry Z. Muller, *The Tyranny of Metrics* (Princeton, NJ: Princeton University Press, 2018).

10. J. P. Simmons, L. D. Nelson, and U. Simonsohn, "False-Positive Psychology: Undisclosed Flexibility in Data Collection and Analysis Allows Presenting Anything as Significant," *Psychological Science* 22, no. 11 (2011).

11. M. L. Head et al., "The Extent and Consequences of P-Hacking in Science," *PLoS Biology* 13, no. 3 (2015).

12. Head et al., "The Extent and Consequences of P-Hacking in Science."

13. Richard Harris, *How Sloppy Science Creates Worthless Cures, Crushes Hope, and Wastes Billions* (New York: Basic Books, 2017).

14. James C. Zimring, "We're Incentivizing Bad Science," *Scientific American*, October 29, 2019.

15. Monya Baker, "Over Half of Psychology Studies Fail Reproducibility Test," *Nature News*, August 27, 2015, 2, https://www.nature.com/articles/nature.2015.18248.

16. This is an informal description of a common approach that was classically defined by John Stuart Mill and is referred to as one of Mill's methods.

17. In real-world analysis, both positive and negative correlates would be analyzed, and a different method may be used to calculate *p* value, but the same general problem would persist.

18. This saying is often called "Hanlon's razor" and has been attributed to multiple sources and in different versions.

11. How Misperceiving Probability Can Be Advantageous

1. For this discussion, I focus on the theory of evolution by natural selection; however, the context of evolution is not required for the findings of cognitive psychology to give rise to contradiction. For someone who holds intelligent design theory to be true, it raises

the question: "Did the designer choose to create us as stupid beings with a flawed ability to reason logically, and if so, why?" However, this theological debate is well outside the scope of the current book.

2. Of course, evolution by natural selection is far more complex. It is not enough for a new trait just to produce more viable offspring, but the offspring must themselves be viable and also be able to generate new viable offspring, and so on. For a trait to be adaptive, the population of increased offspring must have a net viability over time—in other words, traits that lead to such rapid reproduction that populations outgrow their resources and then all die because of overcrowding (e.g., famine) will be selected against. The traits that emerge are those that are best adapted to the environmental specifics that exist. Of course, as the environment changes (as it clearly does), then the traits that are advantageous also will change.

3. H. Mercier and D. Sperber, *The Enigma of Reason* (Cambridge, MA: Harvard University Press, 2017).

4. Z. Kunda, "The Case for Motivated Reasoning," *Psychological Bulletin* 108, no. 3 (1990).

5. S. Frederick, "Cognitive Reflection and Decision Making," *Journal of Economic Perspectives* 19, no. 4 (2005).

6. Harry Markowitz, "Portfolio Selection," *Journal of Finance* 7, no. 1 (1952).

7. G. Gigerenzer, "Heuristics That Make Us Smart" (paper presented at the World Minds Annual Symposium, Zurich, December 2011).

8. This is a model calculation made to test the two approaches in a theoretical situation. The exact number of years of data needed can change based on the number of investment options and the amount of predictive uncertainty. Within these parameters, however, this calculation holds.

9. Note that there are challenges to the dual process theory that question whether System 1 and System 2 are fundamentally different. It has been argued that Systems 1 and 2 are identical in form, because they both are intuitive cognitive modules. System 1 has intuitions about specific things and system 2 has intuitions about reasons; both are the same type of inferential module and focus only on different entities. It has also been argued that System 2's function is not reflective reasoning about the world, but rather it evolved a function in social interactions between humans to provide reasons to explain or justify actions. The fine details of these arguments are outside the scope of this book. It is a fascinating area of cognitive theory, which the interested reader is encouraged to explore. See Mercier and Sperber, *The Enigma of Reason*.

10. H. Garavan, M. E. Doherty, and C. R. Mynatt, "When Falsification Fails," *Irish Journal of Psychology* 18, no. 3 (1997).

11. L. H. Kern, H. L. Mirels, and V. G. Hinshaw, "Scientists' Understanding of Propositional Logic: An Experimental Investigation," *Social Studies of Science* 13, no. 1 (1983).

12. A number of books are devoted to litanies of scientific failures overtime. An excellent work on this topic is W. Gratzer, *The Undergrowth of Science: Delusion, Self-Deception and Human Frailty* (Oxford: Oxford University Press, 2000).

13. Mercier and Sperber, *The Enigma of Reason*.

14. To be fair to Pauling, there is still controversy around use of vitamin C to treat cancer, with some studies showing an effect and others not. There are also findings, however, that vitamin C may promote cancer in other settings. Effects may be related to timing and dose or may just be statistical noise. If anything, this is a testament to the complexity of the real world.

15. L. Cosmides, "The Logic of Social Exchange: Has Natural Selection Shaped How Humans Reason? Studies with the Wason Selection Task," *Cognition* 31, no. 3 (1989); G.

Gigerenzer and K. Hug, "Domain-Specific Reasoning: Social Contracts, Cheating, and Perspective Change," *Cognition* 43, no. 2 (1992); R. S. Nickerson, "Confirmation Bias: A Ubiquitous Phenomenon in Many Guises," *Review of General Psychology* 2, no. 2 (1998).

16. Mercier and Sperber, *The Enigma of Reason.*

17. K. Manktelow, *Reasoning and Thinking* (East Sussex, UK: Psychology Press, 1999), loc. 177 of 4,699, Kindle.

18. There are variations on the exact cards that are shown, but the overall effect is the same.

19. L. Cosmides and J. Tooby, "Adaptations for Reasoning About Social Exchange," in *The Handbook of Evolutionary Psychology*, ed. D. M. Buss (Hoboken, NJ: Wiley, 2015).

20. J. S. B. T. Evans, "Interpretation and Matching Bias in a Reasoning Task," *Quarterly Journal of Experimental Psychology* 24, no. 2 (1972).

21. Cosmides and Tooby, "Adaptations for Reasoning About Social Exchange."

22. Cosmides and Tooby, "Adaptations for Reasoning About Social Exchange."

23. Mercier and Sperber, *The Enigma of Reason*, 4. The *Enigma of Reason* attempts to reconcile not only the question of why have humans been so successful if their reason is so flawed, but also the question of how reason could have evolved as an amazing cognitive addition unrelated to other traits. This latter question is not relevant to the current work, but an excellent argument is presented that reason is an incremental advance in inferential modules that is highly related to more primitive inferential models. Therefore, it is in line with typical patterns of evolutionary development. In doing so, Mercier and Sperber reject dual process theory, the notion that fast thinking (rule of thumb heuristics) and slow thinking (reflective reasoning) are fundamentally different processes. Mercier and Sperber do not deny that "fast" and "slow" thinking exist—their theory encompasses the existing data on these cognitive processes—but they reject the notion that fast and slow thinking are fundamentally different things. Rather, they argue that fast thinking is an inferential module that evaluates environmental experience and slow thinking (reflective reasoning) is an inferential module that evaluates reasons. Both are inferential modules but work on different inputs.

24. The arguments put forth in *The Enigma of Reason* are far more nuanced and complex than can be summarized here. Among other things, the utilities of reason are extended to social constructs in which people use reason to evaluate the arguments of others as well as to justify oneself to others. It is a complex topic, and I highly recommend the interested reader pick up this excellent book. Mercier and Sperber, *The Enigma of Reason.*

25. D. Moshman and M. Geil, "Collaborative Reasoning: Evidence for Collective Rationality," *Thinking and Reasoning* 4, no. 3 (1998).

26. H. Mercier, M. Deguchi, J. B. Van der Henst, and H. Yama, "The Benefits of Argumentation Are Cross-Culturally Robust; the Case of Japan," *Thinking and Reasoning* 22, no. 1 (2016).

27. Moshman and Geil, "Collaborative Reasoning."

28. Mercier and Sperber, *The Enigma of Reason.*

29. N. Oreskes, *Why Trust Science?* (Princeton, NJ: Princeton University Press, 2019), loc. 908 of 8,372, Kindle.

30. K. W. Phillips, "How Diversity Works," *Scientific American* 311, no. 4 (2014).

31. K. W. Phillips and D. L. Loyd, "When Surface and Deep-Level Diversity Collide: The Effects on Dissenting Group Members," *Organizational Behavior and Human Decision Process* 99, no. 2 (2006).

32. D. L. Loyd, C. S. Wang, K. W. Phillips, and R. B. Lount, "Social Category Diversity Promotes Premeeting Elaboration: The Role of Relationship Focus," *Organization Science* 24, no. 3 (2013).

33. A. L. Antonio et al., "Effects of Racial Diversity on Complex Thinking in College Students," *Psychological Science* 15, no. 8 (2004); Phillips, "How Diversity Works."

34. E. Mannix and M. A. Neale, "What Differences Make a Difference? The Promise and Reality of Diverse Teams in Organizations," *Psychological Science in the Public Interest* 6, no. 2 (2005), 31.

35. Mannix and Neale, "What Differences Make a Difference?"

36. In fact, a variety of different types of epistemic network models can be used to simulate different types of systems. In general, epistemic networks are based upon the pioneering work of Bala and Goyal. Venkatesh Bala and Sanjeev Goyal, "Learning from Neighbours," *Review of Economic Studies* 65, no. 3 (1998).

37. Cailin O'Connor and James Owen Wetherall, *The Misinformation Age: How False Beliefs Spread* (New Haven, CT: Yale University Press, 2019).

38. Cailin O'Connor and James Owen Wetherall, "Scientific Polarization," *European Journal of Philosophy of Science* 8 (2018).

39. J. O. Weatherall, C. O'Connor, and J. P. Bruner, "How to Beat Science and Influence People: Policymakers and Propaganda in Epistemic Networks," *British Journal for the Philosophy of Science* 71, no. 4 (2020).

40. The information presented herein regarding the tobacco industry is described in the O'Connor and Wetherall, *The Misinformation Age*, but largely comes from the pioneering work of Naomi Oreskes and Erik M. Conway, *Merchants of Doubt: How a Handful of Scientists Obscured the Truth on Issues from Tobacco Smoke to Global Warming* (New York: Bloomsbury, 2019).

41. In my view, there is a regrettable myopic focus on lung cancer as a risk of smoking. Chances of lung cancer are clearly increased by smoking, and it is good and appropriate for people to be concerned about it. However, the suffering and death from emphysema, chronic obstructive pulmonary disease, heart attacks, strokes, and other maladies also caused by smoking is far more profound than lung cancer. This is the availability heuristic at play, and it serves to help the tobacco industry, as the full magnitude of suffering and sickness caused by their products is consistently underestimated by the populace. I am not saying people should not be allowed to smoke nor that tobacco companies should not be allowed to sell their product. If, however, people choose to smoke, then let them choose to do so with an accurate assessment of the risks.

42. I do not mean to imply that the tobacco industry published excellent science. Such is clearly not the case. The point is that by ignoring the denominator and lying by omission, it is possible to promote an erroneous result with high-quality data. As O'Connor and Weatherall point out, when attempting to lie by omission, it is preferable to run many small studies than fewer larger studies, because the former provides a greater amount of studies with incorrect results that one can selectively report. O'Connor and Wetherall, *The Misinformation Age*.

43. Bennett Holman and Justin Bruner, "Experimentation by Industrial Selection," *Philosophy of Science* 84, no. 5 (2017).

44. This argument is also presented by O'Connor and Weatherall in , *The Misinformation Age*.

45. Garavan, Doherty, and Mynatt, "When Falsification Fails."

46. Kevin J. S. Zollman, "The Communication Structure of Epistemic Communities," *Philosophy of Science* 74, no. 5 (2007).

47. Kevin J. S. Zollman, "The Epistemic Benefit of Transient Diversity," *Erkenntnis* 72, no. 1 (2010).

12. Can Problems with Human Perception and Reasoning Be Solved and Is It Wise to Even Try?

1. D. T. Willingham, "Critical Thinking; Why Is It So Hard to Teach?," *American Educator* 31 (2007), 8.
2. S. O. Lilienfeld, R. Ammirati, and K. Landfield, "Giving Debiasing Away: Can Psychological Research on Correcting Cognitive Errors Promote Human Welfare?," *Perspectives on Psychological Science* 4, no. 4 (2009).
3. H. Arkes, "Costs and Benefits of Judgment Errors: Implications for Debiasing," *Psychological Bulletin* 110, no. 3 (1991).
4. Naïve realism has distinct meanings in the context of philosophy versus psychology; the latter context is being used here.
5. Lilienfeld, Ammirati, and Landfield, "Giving Debiasing Away"; L. Ross and A. Ward, "Naive Realism in Everyday Life: Implications for Social Conflict and Misunderstanding," in *The Jean Piaget Symposium Series. Values and Knowledge*, ed. E. S. Reed, E. Turiel, and T. Brown (Hillsdale, NJ: Lawrence Erlbaum, 1996) , 103–35.
6. Lilienfeld, Ammirati, and Landfield, "Giving Debiasing Away."
7. Lilienfeld, Ammirati, and Landfield, "Giving Debiasing Away."
8. E. Pronin, T. Gilovich, and L. Ross, "Objectivity in the Eye of the Beholder: Divergent Perceptions of Bias in Self Versus Others," *Psychological Review* 111, no. 3 (2004).
9. H. R. Arkes, "Impediments to Accurate Clinical Judgment and Possible Ways to Minimize Their Impact," *Journal of Consulting and Clinical Psychology* 49, no. 3 (1981), 326.
10. Lilienfeld, Ammirati, and Landfield, "Giving Debiasing Away."
11. Willingham, "Critical Thinking," 10.
12. P. W. Cheng, K. J. Holyoak, R. E. Nisbett, and L. M. Oliver, "Pragmatic Versus Syntactic Approaches to Training Deductive Reasoning," *Cognitive Psychology* 18, no. 3 (1986).
13. Willingham, "Critical Thinking"; D. T. Willingham, "How to Teach Critical Thinking," in *Education Future Frontiers* (Department of Education, State of New South Wales, Australia, 2019).
14. Willingham, "Critical Thinking," 8.
15. Willingham, "Critical Thinking," 13.
16. Willingham, "How to Teach Critical Thinking."
17. G. Gigerenzer and U. Hoffrage, "How to Improve Bayesian Reasoning without Instruction: Frequency Formats," *Psychological Review* 102 (1995); P. Weber, K. Binder, and S. Krauss, "Why Can Only 24% Solve Bayesian Reasoning Problems in Natural Frequencies: Frequency Phobia in Spite of Probability Blindness," *Frontiers in Psychology* 9 (2018).
18. The question being asked is, of all the people who happen to have fresh needle pricks, how many of them are addicted to heroin? The answer to this question is a fraction. The top of the fraction is the number of people who have needle pricks and are addicted to heroin, the bottom of the fraction is all of the people who have needle pricks (addicted and nonaddicted). It is important to recognize that all of the people who do not have fresh needle pricks are entirely irrelevant to this question. So, what do we know about the people who *do* have fresh needle pricks? Well, we know that 10 out of 100,000 people (0.01 percent) are heroin addicts and that all of these people will also have fresh needle pricks, because all addicts do. We also know that 190 people (0.19 percent) have fresh needle pricks but are not heroin addicts. So, of all the people who have fresh needle pricks, the fraction of those who are actually heroin addicts is 10 / (10 + 190) = 10 / 200 = ten out of two hundred = one out of twenty (or 5 percent). This type of question is

central to understanding medical diagnosis. If you have a positive test for a disease, how likely are you to actually have the disease? It depends not only on the characteristics of the test but also the frequency of the disease in the population. Even highly trained physicians often fail to answer this question correctly, which shows the difficulty humans tend to have with this type of question. A more detailed discussion of this issue can be found in my book *What Science Is and How It Really Works*, (Cambridge: Cambridge University Press, 2019), 192–95.

19. M. McDowell and P. Jacobs, "Meta-Analysis of the Effect of Natural Frequencies on Bayesian Reasoning," *Psychological Bulletin* 143, no. 12 (2017).

20. Weber, Binder, and Krauss, "Why Can Only 24% Solve Bayesian Reasoning Problems in Natural Frequencies," 1.

21. Weber, Binder, and Krauss, "Why Can Only 24% Solve Bayesian Reasoning Problems in Natural Frequencies," 11.

22. B. Swire-Thompson, J. DeGutis, and D. Lazer, "Searching for the Backfire Effect: Measurement and Design Considerations," *Journal of Applied Research in Memory and Cognition* 9, no. 3 (2020).

23. Of course, I do not mean to imply that all things have the same probability of happening irrespective of the rules of nature. If one places paper in a flame, the probability of it burning is much higher than the probability of it turning into a bird and flying away. I am speaking rather to more complex events under conditions of uncertainty.

24. Robert B. Stinnett, *Day of Deceit: The Truth About FDR and Pearl Harbor* (New York: Free Press, 2000).

25. "Testimony of Condoleezza Rice Before 9/11 Commission," *New York Times*, April 8, 2004.

26. "Bin Ladin Determined to Strike in US," National Security Archive, August 6, 2001, Central Intelligence Agency, declassified and approved for release, April 10, 2004, https://irp.fas.org/cia/product/pdb080601.pdf.

27. L. J. Sanna, N. Schwarz, and S. L. Stocker, "When Debiasing Backfires: Accessible Content and Accessibility Experiences in Debiasing Hindsight," *Journal of Experimental Psychology: Learning, Memory, and Cognition* 28, no. 3 (2002).

28. Comparing two groups of participants instructed to imagine two versus ten different outcomes, respectively, was chosen based on a prestudy survey that established a subjective feeling of difficulty in thinking of ten different outcomes, but no such feeling with only two different outcomes.

29. P. M. Fernbach, T. Rogers, C. R. Fox, and S. A. Sloman, "Political Extremism Is Supported by an Illusion of Understanding," *Psychological Science* 24, no. 6 (2013).

30. L. Rozenblit and F. Keil, "The Misunderstood Limits of Folk Science: An Illusion of Explanatory Depth," *Cognitive Science* 26, no. 5 (2002).

31. Eli Pariser, *The Filter Bubble: How the New Personalized Web Is Changing What We Read and How We Think* (London: Penguin, 2011).

32. D. Geschke, J. Lorenz, and P. Holtz, "The Triple-Filter Bubble: Using Agent-Based Modelling to Test a Meta-Theoretical Framework for the Emergence of Filter Bubbles and Echo Chambers," *British Journal of Social Psychology* 58, no. 1 (2019), 129.

33. On an editorial note, I am not a researcher in these fields, and I would not benefit directly, professionally, or personally from more support for research in these areas.

BIBLIOGRAPHY

Al-Lamee, R., D. Thompson, H. M. Dehbi, S. Sen, K. Tang, J. Davies, T. Keeble, et al. "Percutaneous Coronary Intervention in Stable Angina (Orbita): A Double-Blind, Randomised Controlled Trial." *Lancet* 391, no. 10115 (2018): 31–40.

Althaus, Scott L. and Devon M. Largio. "When Osama Became Saddam: Origins and Consequences of the Change in America's Public Enemy #1." *PS: Political Science and Politics* 37, no. 4 (2004): 795–99.

An, S. "Antidepressant Direct-to-Consumer Advertising and Social Perception of the Prevalence of Depression: Application of the Availability Heuristic." *Health Communication* 23, no. 6 (2008): 499–505.

Antonio, A. L., M. J. Chang, K. Hakuta, D. A. Kenny, S. Levin, and J. F. Milem. "Effects of Racial Diversity on Complex Thinking in College Students." *Psychological Science* 15, no. 8 (2004): 507–10.

Arkes, H. "Costs and Benefits of Judgment Errors: Implications for Debiasing." *Psychological Bulletin* 110, no. 3 (1991): 486–98.

——. "Impediments to Accurate Clinical Judgment and Possible Ways to Minimize Their Impact." *Journal of Consulting and Clinical Psychology* 49, no. 3 (1981): 323–30.

Bagley, C., and P. Tremblay. "Elevated Rates of Suicidal Behavior in Gay, Lesbian, and Bisexual Youth." *Crisis* 21, no. 3 (2000): 111–7.

Baker, Monya. "Over Half of Psychology Studies Fail Reproducibility Test." *Nature News*, August 27, 2015. https://www.nature.com/articles/nature.2015.18248.

Baker, Peter. "Trump Pardons Scooter Libby in a Case That Mirrors His Own." *New York Times*, April 13, 2018.

Baker, Peter, and Michael Cooper. "In Romney and Obama Speeches, Selective Truths." *New York Times*, June 19, 2012.

Bala, Venkatesh, and Sanjeev Goyal. "Learning from Neighbours." *Review of Economic Studies* 65, no. 3 (1998): 595–621.

Bar-Hillel, M., D. Bar-Natan, and B. McKay. "Solving the Bible Code Puzzle." *Statistical Science* 14 (1999): 150–73.

Baron, J. "Myside Bias in Thinking About Abortion." *Thinking and Reasoning* 1, no. 3 (1995): 221–35.

Barr, Jeremy. "Axios's Jonathan Swan Is the Latest Interviewer to Leave Trump Gasping on TV." *Washington Post*, August 4, 2020.

Bering, Jesse. *The Belief Instinct: The Psychology of Souls, Destiny, and the Meaning of Life.* New York: Norton, 2011.

"Bin Ladin Determined to Strike in US." National Security Archive, August 6, 2001. Central Intelligence Agency, declassified and approved for release, April 10, 2004. https://irp.fas.org/cia/product/pdb080601.pdf.

Boulware, D. R., M. F. Pullen, A. S. Bangdiwala, K. A. Pastick, S. M. Lofgren, E. C. Okafor, C. P. Skipper, et al. "A Randomized Trial of Hydroxychloroquine as Postexposure Prophylaxis for Covid-19." *New England Journal of Medicine* 383, no. 6 (2020): 517–25.

"Brandon Mroz Lands Historic Quad Lutz." *ESPN*, November 12, 2011. https://www.espn.com/olympics/figureskating/story/_/id/7223251/brandon-mroz-makes-skating-history-quadruple-lutz-nhk-trophy.

Bruner, J. S., and M. C. Potter. "Interference in Visual Recognition." *Science* 144, no. 3617 (1964): 424–5.

Buerkel-Rothfuss, N. L., and S. Mayes. "Soap Opera Viewing: The Cultivation Effect." *Journal of Communication* 31, no. 3 (1981): 108–15.

Bump, Philip. "Trump's Stunning Claim That He's Taking Hydroxychloroquine Could Trigger a Cascade of Negative Effects." *Washington Post*, May 18, 2020.

Burns, Alexander. "Choice Words from Donald Trump, Presidential Candidate." *New York Times*, June 16, 2015.

Butcher, Kristin F., and Anne Morrison Piehl. "Crime, Corrections, and California: What Does Immigration Have to Do with It?" *Public Policy Institute of California Population Trends and Profiles* 9, no. 3 (2008).

California State Auditor. "The CalGant Criminal Intelligence System Report." Report 2015-130, Sacramento, California, August 2016.

Chabria, Anita, Kevin Rector, and C. Chang. "California Bars Police from Using LAPD Records in Gang Database. Critics Want It Axed." *Los Angeles Times*, July 14, 2020.

Chabris, Christopher, and Daniel Simons. *The Invisible Gorilla: How Our Intuitions Deceive Us.* New York: Crown Publishing, 2009.

Cheney, Richard. "Cheney on Bin Laden Tape." By Tim Russert. *Meet the Press*, NBC, December 9, 2001.

Cheng, P. W., K. J. Holyoak, R. E. Nisbett, and L. M. Oliver. "Pragmatic Versus Syntactic Approaches to Training Deductive Reasoning." *Cognitive Psychology* 18, no. 3 (1986): 293–328.

Cherney, A. "The Effect of Common Features on Brand Choice: Moderating the Effect of Attribute Importance." *Journal of Consumer Research* 23 (1997): 304–11.

Chulov, Martin, and Helen Pidd. "Curveball: How US Was Duped by Iraqi Fantasist Looking to Topple Saddam." *Guardian*, February 15, 2011.

Churchland, Patricia S., V. S. Ramachandran, and Terrence J. Sejnowski. "A Critique of Pure Vision." In *Large Scale Neuronal Theories of the Brain*, ed. Christof Koch and Joel L. Davis, 23–60. Cambridge, MA: MIT Press, 1994.

"Citrus Christ? Cheesus? 13 Religious Sightings: God Is Everywhere-Including an Orange, a Cat's Fur and a Bag of Cheetos." *Today*, July 20, 2011. http://www.today.com/id/39750888/ns/today-today_news/t/citrus-christ-cheesus-religious-sightings/#.XlvWbnwo6Ul.

Cosmides, L. "The Logic of Social Exchange: Has Natural Selection Shaped How Humans Reason? Studies with the Wason Selection Task." *Cognition* 31, no. 3 (1989): 187–276.

Cosmides, L., and J. Tooby. "Adaptations for Reasoning About Social Exchange." In *The Handbook of Evolutionary Psychology*, ed. D. M. Buss, 625–28. Hoboken, NJ: Wiley, 2015.

Creators Syndicate. "The CIA Leak." *CNN Inside Politics*, CNN, October 1, 2003.

Cruz, Ted. "One-on-One Interview with Ted Cruz." By Jay Root, *Texas Tribune*, March 25, 2015. https://www.texastribune.org/2015/03/24/livestream-one-on-one-interview-with-ted -cruz/

——. "Scientific Evidence Doesn't Support Global Warming, Sen. Ted Cruz Says." By Steve Inskeep and David Greene. *Morning Edition*, NPR, December 9, 2015.

Davies, Paul. *The Goldilocks Enigma: Why Is the Universe Just Right for Life?* London: Allen Lane, 2006.

de Wit, J. B. F., E. Das, and R. Vet. "What Works Best: Objective Statistics or a Personal Testimonial? An Assessment of the Persuasive Effects of Different Types of Message Evidence on Risk Perception." *Health Psychology* 27, no. 1 (2008): 110–15.

Dear, William. *The Dungeon Master: The Disappearance of James Dallas Egbert III.* Boston: Houghton Mifflin, 1984.

Dembski, William A. *The Design Inference: Eliminating Chance Through Small Probabilities.* Cambridge Studies in Probability, Induction and Decision Theory. Cambridge: Cambridge University Press, 1998.

Draper, R. *To Start a War: How the Bush Administration Took America into Iraq.* New York: Penguin, 2020.

Drosnin, Michael. *The Bible Code.* New York: Touchstone, 1998.

Dutton, Kevin. *Black and White Thinking: The Burden of a Binary Brain in a Complex World.* London: Bantam, 2020.

Editorial Board. "Who Will Kill or Be Killed in Violence-Plagued Chicago? The Algorithm Knows." *Chicago Tribune*, May 10, 2016.

Edward, Mark. "The Clown in the Graveyard." *Skeptical Inquirer*, April 20, 2016. https://skeptical inquirer.org/exclusive/the-clown-in-the-graveyard/.

Evans, J. S. B. T. "Interpretation and Matching Bias in a Reasoning Task." *Quarterly Journal of Experimental Psychology* 24, no. 2 (1972): 193–99.

——. "Reasoning, Biases and Dual Processes: The Lasting Impact of Wason (1960)." *Quarterly Journal of Experimental Psychology* 69, no. 10 (2016): 2076–92.

"Excess Deaths Associated with Covid-19." Centers for Disease Control and Prevention, National Center for Health Statistics. Last reviewed November 6, 2015. https://www.cdc .gov/nchs/nvss/vsrr/covid19/excess_deaths.htm accessed 9-19-2020.

Ferguson, Andrew Gutherie. *The Rise of Big Data Policing: Surveillance, Race and the Future of Law Enforcement.* New York: New York University Press, 2017.

Ferguson, C. J. "Evidence for Publication Bias in Video Game Violence Effects Literature: A Meta-Analytic Review." *Aggression and Violent Behavior* 12, no. 4 (2007): 470–82.

Fernbach, P. M., T. Rogers, C. R. Fox, and S. A. Sloman. "Political Extremism Is Supported by an Illusion of Understanding." *Psychological Science* 24, no. 6 (2013): 939–46.

Frederick, S. "Cognitive Reflection and Decision Making." *Journal of Economic Perspectives* 19, no. 4 (2005): 25–42.

"Frequently Asked Questions." Centers for Disease Control and Prevention. Last reviewed November 26, 2019. https://www.cdc.gov/plague/faq/index.html.

Garavan, H., M. E. Doherty, and C. R. Mynatt. "When Falsification Fails." *Irish Journal of Psychology* 18, no. 3 (1997): 267–92.

German, Mike. *Disrupt, Discredit and Divide: How the New FBI Damages Democracy.* New York: New Press, 2019.

Geschke, D., J. Lorenz, and P. Holtz. "The Triple-Filter Bubble: Using Agent-Based Modelling to Test a Meta-Theoretical Framework for the Emergence of Filter Bubbles and Echo Chambers." *British Journal of Social Psychology* 58, no. 1 (2019): 129–49.

Gigerenzer, G. "Heuristics That Make Us Smart." Paper presented at the World Minds Annual Symposium, Zurich, December 2011.

Gigerenzer, G., and U. Hoffrage. "How to Improve Bayesian Reasoning without Instruction: Frequency Formats." *Psychological Review* 102 (1995): 684–703

Gigerenzer, G., and K. Hug. "Domain-Specific Reasoning: Social Contracts, Cheating, and Perspective Change." *Cognition* 43, no. 2 (1992): 127–71.

Gopnik, A. "Explanation as Orgasm and the Drive for Causal Understanding: The Evolution, Function, and Phenomenology of the Theory-Formation System." In *Cognition and Explanation*, ed. F. Keil and R. Wilson, 299–323. Cambridge, MA: MIT Press, 2000.

Gorman, Sara E., and Jack M. Gorman. *Denying to the Grave: Why We Ignore the Facts That Will Save Us.* New York: Oxford University Press, 2017.

Gratzer, W. *The Undergrowth of Science: Delusion, Self-Deception and Human Frailty.* Oxford: Oxford University Press, 2000.

Green, Elizabeth. "Why Do Americans Stink at Math?" *New York Times Magazine*, July 23, 2014.

Griffiths, Mark, and Richard Wood. "The Psychology of Lottery Gambling." *International Gambling Studies* 1, no. 1 (2001): 27–45.

Haberman, Clyde. "When Dungeons & Dragons Set Off a 'Moral Panic.' " *New York Times Retro Report*, April 17, 2016.

Hansen, J., R. Ruedy, M. Sato, and K. Lo. "Global Surface Temperature Change." *Review of Geophysics* 48, no. 4 (2010): RG4004.

Harris, Richard. *How Sloppy Science Creates Worthless Cures, Crushes Hope, and Wastes Billions.* New York: Basic Books, 2017.

Head, M. L., L. Holman, R. Lanfear, A. T. Kahn, and M. D. Jennions. "The Extent and Consequences of P-Hacking in Science." *PLoS Biology* 13, no. 3 (2015): e1002106.

Hertz, Noreena. *Eyes Wide Open: How to Make Smart Decisions in a Confusing World.* New York: HarperCollins, 2013.

Holman, Bennett, and Justin Bruner. "Experimentation by Industrial Selection." *Philosophy of Science* 84, no. 5 (2017): 1008–19.

Hoyle, Fred. "The Universe: Past and Present Reflections." *Engineering and Science Magazine*, November 1981, 8–12.

Jehl, Douglas. "Qaeda-Iraq Link U.S. Cited Is Tied to Coercion Claim." *New York Times*, December 9, 2005.

Johnson, Jenna. " 'A Lot of People Are Saying . . .': How Trump Spreads Conspiracies and Innuendoes." *Washington Post*, June 13, 2016.

Kahneman, Daniel, and Frederick Shane. "Representativeness Revisted: Attribute Substitution in Intuitive Judgement." In *Heuristics and Biases: The Psychology of Intuitive Judgment*, ed. Thomas Gilovich, Dale Griffin, and Daniel Kahneman, 49–81. Cambridge, UK: Cambridge University Press, 2002.

Kahneman, Daniel, Paul Slovic, and Amos Tversky. *Judgement under Uncertainty: Heuristics and Biases.* London: Cambridge University Press, 1982.

Kampourakis, Kostas. *Understanding Evolution.* Cambridge: Cambridge University Press, 2020.

Kask, T. J. "Dragon Rumbles." *The Dragon*, October 1979.

Kazoleas, Dean C. "A Comparison of the Persuasive Effectiveness of Qualitative Versus Quantitative Evidence. A Test of Explanatory Hypotheses." *Communications Quarterly* 41, no. 1 (1993): 40–50.

Kern, L. H., H. L. Mirels, and V. G. Hinshaw. "Scientists' Understanding of Propositional Logic: An Experimental Investigation." *Social Studies of Science* 13, no. 1 (1983): 131–46.

Kessler, Glenn. "Valerie Plame's Claim That Scooter Libby Leaked Her Identity." *Washington Post*, September 10, 2019.

Klein, J. G. "Five Pitfalls in Decisions About Diagnosis and Prescribing." *British Medical Journal* 330, no. 7494 (2005): 781–3.

Koehler, J. J. "One in Millions, Billions, and Trillions: Lessons from People V. Collins (1968) for People V. Simpson (1995)." *Journal of Legal Education* 147, no. 2 (June 1997): 214–23.

Kunda, Z. "The Case for Motivated Reasoning." *Psychological Bulletin* 108, no. 3 (1990): 480–98.

Lehrer, Tom. "Dialog." Track 11, "We Will All Go Together When We Go." On *An Evening Wasted with Tom Lehrer*. Warner Bros Records, 1959.

Leslie, John. *Universes*. London: Routledge, 1989.

Levitan, D. *Not a Scientist: How Politicians Mistake, Misrepresent, and Utterly Mangle Science*. New York: Norton, 2017.

Lichtblau, Eric. "2002 Memo Doubted Uranium Sale Claim." *New York Times*, January 18, 2006.

Lilienfeld, S. O., R. Ammirati, and K. Landfield. "Giving Debiasing Away: Can Psychological Research on Correcting Cognitive Errors Promote Human Welfare?" *Perspectives on Psychological Science* 4, no. 4 (Jul 2009): 390–8.

Lind, M., M. Visentini, T. Mantyla, and F. Del Missier. "Choice-Supportive Misremembering: A New Taxonomy and Review." *Frontiers in Psychology* 8 (2017): 2062.

Lipton, Peter. *Inference to the Best Explanation*. 2nd ed. International Library of Philosophy. London: Routledge, 2004.

Lord, C. G., L. Ross, and M. R. Lepper. "Biased Assimilation and Attitude Polarization. The Effects of Prior Theories on Subsequently Considered Evidence." *Journal of Personality and Social Psychology* 37, no. 11 (1979): 2098–109.

Loyd, D. L., C. S. Wang, K. W. Phillips, and R. B. Lount. "Social Category Diversity Promotes Premeeting Elaboration: The Role of Relationship Focus." *Organization Science* 24, no. 3 (2013): 757–72.

Mangel, M., and F. J. Samaniego. "Abraham Wald's Work on Aircraft Survivability." *Journal of American Statistical Association* 79, no. 386 (1984): 259–67.

Manktelow, K. *Reasoning and Thinking*. East Sussex, UK: Psychology Press, 1999.

Mannix, E., and M. A. Neale. "What Differences Make a Difference? The Promise and Reality of Diverse Teams in Organizations." *Psychological Science in the Public Interest* 6, no. 2 (2005): 31–55.

Markowitz, Harry. "Portfolio Selection." *Journal of Finance* 7, no. 1 (1952): 77–91.

Matthews, Jeffrey J. *Colin Powell: Imperfect Patriot*. Notre Dame, IN: University of Notre Dame Press, 2019.

McConkie, G. W., and K. Rayner. "The Span of Effective Stimulus During a Fixation in Reading." *Perception and Psychophysics* 17, no. 6 (1975): 578–86.

McDowell, M., and P. Jacobs. "Meta-Analysis of the Effect of Natural Frequencies on Bayesian Reasoning." *Psychological Bulletin* 143, no. 12 (2017): 1273–312.

McIntyre, Lee. *Post-Truth*. Cambridge, MA: MIT Press, 2018.

——. *The Scientific Attitude: Defending Science from Denial, Fraud, and Pseudoscience*. Cambridge, MA: MIT Press, 2019.

McLaren, Karla. "Bridging the Chasm Between Two Cultures." *Skeptical Inquirer* 28, no. 3 (2004): 47–52.

Mercier, H. "Confirmation Bias-Myside Bias." In *Cognitive Illusions: Intriguing Phenomena in Thinking, Judgment and Memory*, ed. R. F. Pohl, 99–114. London: Routledge, 2017.

Mercier, H., M. Deguchi, J. B. Van der Henst, and H. Yama. "The Benefits of Argumentation Are Cross-Culturally Robust; the Case of Japan." *Thinking and Reasoning* 22, no. 1 (2016): 1–15.

Mercier, H., and D. Sperber. *The Enigma of Reason*. Cambridge, MA: Harvard University Press, 2017.

Meyer, Stephen C. *The Return of the God Hypothesis: Compelling Scientific Evidence for the Existence of God*. New York: HarperOne, 2020.

Miller, G. A. *The Psychology of Communication*. New York: Basic Books, 1967.

Moshman, D., and M. Geil. "Collaborative Reasoning: Evidence for Collective Rationality." *Thinking and Reasoning* 4, no. 3 (1998): 231–48.

Muller, Jerry Z. *The Tyranny of Metrics*. Princeton, NJ: Princeton University Press, 2018.

Mylroie, Laurie. *Study of Revenge: Saddam Hussein's Unfinished War Against America*. Washington, DC: AIE Press, 2000.

National Safety Council of America. "Odds of Dying." https://injuryfacts.nsc.org/all-injuries/preventable-death-overview/odds-of-dying/?

Nichols, Michelle. "Ex-CIA Chief Says 'Slam Dunk' Iraq Quote Misused." *Reuters*, April 26, 2007.

Nickerson, R. S. "Confirmation Bias: A Ubiquitous Phenomenon in Many Guises." *Review of General Psychology* 2, no. 2 (1998): 175–220.

Nostradamus. *The Complete Prophecies of Nostradamus*. New York: Start Publishing, 2012.

Nowrasteh, Alex. "Immigration and Crime—What the Research Says." *Cato at Library* (blog), June 14, 2015. https://www.cato.org/blog/immigration-crime-what-research-says.

——. "The White House's Misleading & Error Ridden Narrative on Immigrants and Crime." *Cato at Library* (blog), June 25, 2018. https://www.cato.org/blog/white-houses-misleading-error-ridden-narrative-immigrants-crime.

O'Connor, Cailin, and James Owen Weatherall. "Scientific Polarization." *European Journal of Philosophy of Science* 8 (2018): 855–75.

——. *The Misinformation Age: How False Beliefs Spread*. New Haven, CT: Yale University Press, 2019.

O'Guinn, T. C., and L. J. Shrum. "The Role of Television in the Construction of Consumer Reality." *Journal of Consumer Research* 23 (1997): 278–94.

Oreskes, Naomi. *Why Trust Science?* Princeton, NJ: Princeton University Press, 2019.

Oreskes, Naomi, and Erik M. Conway. *Merchants of Doubt: How a Handful of Scientists Obscured the Truth on Issues from Tobacco Smoke to Global Warming*. New York: Bloomsbury, 2019.

Paley, William. *Natural Theology, or, Evidences of the Existence and Attributes of the Deity, Collected from the Appearances of Nature*. London: R. Faulder, 1803.

Pammer, K., S. Sabadas, and S. Lentern. "Allocating Attention to Detect Motorcycles: The Role of Inattentional Blindness." *Human Factors* 60, no. 1 (2018): 5–19.

Pariser, Eli. *The Filter Bubble: How the New Personalized Web Is Changing What We Read and How We Think*. London: Penguin, 2011.

Paulos, John A. *Innumeracy: Mathematical Illiteracy and Its Consequences*. New York: Hill and Wang, 2001.

Penrose, Roger. *The Emperor's New Mind: Concerning Computers, Minds, and the Laws of Physics*. Oxford: Oxford University Press, 1989.

People V. Collins, 438, P.2d 33, 34 (Cal. 1968) (1968).

Perez-Pena, Richard. "Contrary to Trump's Claims, Immigrants Are Less Likely to Commit Crimes." *New York Times*, January 26, 2017.

Peterson, C. R., and W. M. DuCharme. "A Primacy Effect in Subjective Probability Revision." *Journal of Experimental Psychology* 73, no. 1 (1967): 61–5.

Peterson, Jon. *Playing at the World: A History of Simulating Wars, People and Fantastic Adventures, from Chess to Role-Playing Games*. San Diego, CA: Unreason Press, 2012.

Phillips, K. W. "How Diversity Works." *Scientific American* 311, no. 4 (2014): 42–7.

Phillips, K. W., and D. L. Loyd. "When Surface and Deep-Level Diversity Collide: The Effects on Dissenting Group Members." *Organizational Behavior and Human Decision Process* 99, no. 2 (2006): 143–60.

Pitz, G. F., L. Downing, and H. Reinhold. "Sequential Effects in the Revision of Subjective Probabilities." *Canadian Journal of Psychology* 21 (1967): 381–93.

Poses, R. M., and M. Anthony. "Availability, Wishful Thinking, and Physicians' Diagnostic Judgments for Patients with Suspected Bacteremia." *Medical Decision Making* 11, no. 3 (1991): 159–68.

Pronin, E., T. Gilovich, and L. Ross. "Objectivity in the Eye of the Beholder: Divergent Perceptions of Bias in Self Versus Others." *Psychological Review* 111, no. 3 (2004): 781–99.

Rappeport, Allan, and Alexander Burns. "Donald Trump Says He Will Accept Election Outcome ('If I Win')." *New York Times*, October 20, 2016.

Rice, Condoleezza. By Wolf Blitzer. *CNN Late Edition with Wolf Blitzer*, CNN, September 8, 2002.

Rosenbaum, David E. "A Closer Look at Cheney and Halliburton." *New York Times*, September 28, 2004.

Rosenberg, Matthew. "Afghan Sign of Progress Turns out to Be Error." *New York Times*, February 26, 2013.

Ross, L., and A. Ward. "Naive Realism in Everyday Life: Implications for Social Conflict and Misunderstanding." In *The Jean Piaget Symposium Series. Values and Knowledge*, ed. E. S. Reed, E. Turiel, and T. Brown, 103–35. Hillsdale, NJ: Lawrence Erlbaum, 1996.

Rozenblit, L., and F. Keil. "The Misunderstood Limits of Folk Science: An Illusion of Explanatory Depth." *Cognitive Science* 26, no. 5 (2002): 521–62.

Rumsfeld, Donald. By Stephen Colbert. *The Late Show with Stephen Colbert*, CBS, January 26, 2016.

Sanna, L. J., N. Schwarz, and S. L. Stocker. "When Debiasing Backfires: Accessible Content and Accessibility Experiences in Debiasing Hindsight." *Journal of Experimental Psychology: Learning, Memory, and Cognition* 28, no. 3 (2002): 497–502.

Schatz, Bryan. "A Former FBI Whistleblower Explains Why the Federal Government Is Failing on Domestic Terrorism—and How to Fix It." *Mother Jones*, August 7, 2019.

Seelye, Katharine Q. "Fraction of Americans with Drug Addiction Receive Treatment, Surgeon General Says." *New York Times*, November 17, 2016.

Self, W. H., M. W. Semler, L. M. Leither, J. D. Casey, D. C. Angus, R. G. Brower, S. Y. Chang, et al. "Effect of Hydroxychloroquine on Clinical Status at 14 Days in Hospitalized Patients with Covid-19: A Randomized Clinical Trial." *Journal of the American Medical Association* 324, no. 21 (2020): 2165–76.

Shanker, Thom "New Strategy Vindicates Ex-Army Chief Shinseki." *New York Times*, January 12, 2007.

"The Share of Covid-19 Tests That Are Positive." Our World in Data, University of Oxford, Oxford Martin School. https://ourworldindata.org/grapher/positive-rate-daily-smoothed?tab=chart&time=earliest..2020-07-28.

Shao, R., and Y. Wang. "The Relation of Violent Video Games to Adolescent Aggression: An Examination of Moderated Mediation Effect." *Frontiers in Psychology* 10 (2019): 384.

Shermer, Michael. *How We Believe: Science, Skepticism, and the Search of God.* New York: W. H. Freeman, 1999.

Simmons, J. P., L. D. Nelson, and U. Simonsohn. "False-Positive Psychology: Undisclosed Flexibility in Data Collection and Analysis Allows Presenting Anything as Significant." *Psychological Science* 22, no. 11 (2011): 1359–66.

Sinclair, Upton. *I, Candidate for Governor: And How I Got Licked.* Berkeley: University of California Press, 1934.

Sloman, Steven A., and Philip Fernback. *The Knowledge Illusion: Why We Never Think Alone.* New York: Riverhead, 2017.

Smith, Gary. *Standard Deviations: Flawed Assumptions, Tortured Data, and Other Ways to Lie with Statistics.* New York: Overlook Duckworth, 2019.

Stenger, Victor J. *The Fallacy of Fine-Tuning: Why the Universe Is Not Designed for Us.* Amherst, NY: Prometheus, 2011.

Stewart, S. T., D. M. Cutler, and A. B. Rosen. "Forecasting the Effects of Obesity and Smoking on U.S. Life Expectancy." *New England Journal of Medicine* 361, no. 23 (2009): 2252–60.

Stinnett, Robert B. *Day of Deceit: The Truth About FDR and Pearl Harbor.* New York: Free Press, 2000.

Stout, David. "Subject of C.I.A. Leak Testifies on Capitol Hill." *New York Times*, March 16, 2007.

Swire-Thompson, B., J. DeGutis, and D. Lazer. "Searching for the Backfire Effect: Measurement and Design Considerations." *Journal of Applied Research in Memory and Cognition* 9, no. 3 (2020): 286–99.

Tenet, George. *At the Center of the Storm: My Years at the CIA.* New York: Harper Luxe, 2007.

"Testimony of Condoleezza Rice Before 9/11 Commission." *New York Times*, April 8, 2004.

Thoreau, Henry David. "Autumnal Tints." *The Atlantic*, 1862.

Thucydides. *History of the Peloponnesian War.* Trans. Rex Warner, ed. M. I. Finley. London: Penguin Classics, 1972.

Tik, M., R. Sladky, C. D. B. Luft, D. Willinger, A. Hoffmann, M. J. Banissy, J. Bhattacharya, and C. Windischberger. "Ultra-High-Field fMRI Insights on Insight: Neural Correlates of the Aha!-Moment." *Human Brain Mapping* 39, no. 8 (2018): 3241–52.

Tuchman, Barbara W. *The March of Folly: From Troy to Vietnam.* New York: Random House, 2014.

Tversky, Amos, and Daniel Kahneman. "Availability: A Heuristic for Judging Frequency and Probability." *Cognitive Psychology* 5, no. 2 (1973): 207–32.

Tweney, R. D., M. E. Doherty, W. J. Warner, D. B. Pliske, C. R. Mynatt, K. A. Gross, and D. L. Arkkelin. "Strategies of Rule Discovery in an Inference Task." *Quarterly Journal of Experimental Psychology* 32 (1980): 109–23.

U.S. Bureau of Labor Statistics. "Labor Force Statistics from the Current Population Survey." https://data.bls.gov/pdq/SurveyOutputServlet.

"U.S. Passenger-Miles." U.S. Department of Transportation Bureau of Transportation Statistics. https://www.bts.gov/content/us-passenger-miles.

Van Dam, Andrew. "The Awful Reason Wages Appeared to Soar in the Middle of a Pandemic." *Washington Post*, May 8, 2020.

Vigen, Tyler. *Spurious Correlations.* New York: Hachette, 2015.

Vincent, M. J., E. Bergeron, S. Benjannet, B. R. Erickson, P. E. Rollin, T. G. Ksiazek, N. G. Seidah, and S. T. Nichol. "Chloroquine Is a Potent Inhibitor of SARS Coronavirus Infection and Spread." *Virology Journal* 2 (2005): 69.

Von Drehle, David, and Jeffrey R. Smit. "U.S. Strikes Iraq for Plot to Kill Bush." *Washington Post*, June 27, 1993.

Wainberg, James. "Stories vs. Statistics: The Impact of Anecdotal Data on Managerial Decision Making." In *Advances in Accounting Behavior Research*, ed. K. E. Karim, 127–42. Bingley, UK: Emerald, 2019.

Wainberg, James, Thomas Kida, and James Smith. "Stories vs. Statistics: The Impact of Anecdotal Data on Professional Decision Making." *SSRN Electronic Journal* (2010). doi:10.2139/ssrn.1571358.

Walliss, John. *The Bloody Code in England and Wales, 1760–1830.* World Histories of Crime, Culture and Violence.,ed. M. Muravyeva and R. M. Tovio. Cham, Switzerland: Palgrave Macmillan, 2018.

Walsh, N. P. "The Lies That Were Told to Sustain the US and UK Mission in Afghanistan." *CNN*, May 30, 2021.

"Washington Post Police Shooting Database." https://www.washingtonpost.com/graphics/investigations/police-shootings-database/.

Wason, P. C. "On the Failure to Eliminate Hypotheses in a Conceptual Task." *Quarterly Journal of Experimental Psychology* 12, no. 3 (1960): 129–40.

Wasserstein, R. L., and N. A. Lazar. "The ASA Statement on *p*-Values: Context, Process, and Purpose." *American Statistician* 70, no. 2 (2016): 129–33.

Weatherall, J. O., C. O'Connor, and J. P. Bruner. "How to Beat Science and Influence People: Policymakers and Propaganda in Epistemic Networks." *British Journal for the Philosophy of Science* 71, no. 4 (2020): 1–30.

Weber, P., K. Binder, and S. Krauss. "Why Can Only 24% Solve Bayesian Reasoning Problems in Natural Frequencies: Frequency Phobia in Spite of Probability Blindness." *Frontiers in Psychology* 9 (2018): 1833.

Westen, D., P. S. Blagov, K. Harenski, C. Kilts, and S. Hamann. "Neural Bases of Motivated Reasoning: An fMRI Study of Emotional Constraints on Partisan Political Judgment in the 2004 U.S. Presidential Election." *Journal of Cognitive Neuroscience* 18, no. 11 (2006): 1947–58.

The White House. President George W. Bush Archives. "President Bush Outlines Iraqi Threat." Office of the Press Secretary, October 7, 2002. https://georgewbush-whitehouse.archives.gov/news/releases/2002/10/20021007-8.html.

Willingham, D. T. "Critical Thinking; Why Is It So Hard to Teach?" *American Educator* 31 (2007): 8–19.

——. "How to Teach Critical Thinking." In *Education Future Frontiers*. Occasional Paper Series. Department of Education, State of New South Wales, Australia, 2019.

Winterbottom, A., H. L. Bekker, M. Conner, and A. Mooney. "Does Narrative Information Bias Individual's Decision Making? A Systematic Review." *Social Science and Medicine* 67, no. 12 (2008): 2079–88.

Wolfowitz, Paul, and Zalmay Khalilzad. "Overthrow Him." *Weekly Standard*, December 1, 1997.

Woodward, Bob. *Plan of Attack.* New York: Simon & Schuster, 2004.

Zimring, James C. "We're Incentivizing Bad Science." *Scientific American*, October 29, 2019.

——. *What Science Is and How It Really Works* (Cambridge: Cambridge University Press, 2019).

Zollman, Kevin J. S. "The Communication Structure of Epistemic Communities." *Philosophy of Science* 74, no. 5 (2007): 574–87.

——. "The Epistemic Benefit of Transient Diversity." *Erkenntnis* 72, no. 1 (2010): 17–35.

INDEX

Page numbers in *italics* indicate figures or tables.